To my radiant stars, Tyan and Aidan,
Your presence has been the compass guiding me to greatness, urging
me to evolve, to learn, and to be the best version of myself. Every
word in this book carries a fragment of the love and inspiration you
both have bestowed upon me. May you always know the depth of
my gratitude and love. This book is a testament to the power you've
granted me.

Get Your Sexy Back

Biohacking Your Menopause Journey

Dr. Chai Ling Low

Copyright © 2023 by Dr. Chai Ling Low

All rights reserved.

No portion of this book may be reproduced in any form without written permission from the publisher or author, except as permitted by U.S. copyright law.

This publication is designed to provide accurate and authoritative information in regard to the subject matter covered. It is sold with the understanding that neither the author nor the publisher is engaged in rendering legal, investment, accounting or other professional services. While the publisher and author have used their best efforts in preparing this book, they make no representations or warranties with respect to the accuracy or completeness of the contents of this book and specifically disclaim any implied warranties of merchantability or fitness for a particular purpose. No warranty may be created or extended by sales representatives or written sales materials. The advice and strategies contained herein may not be suitable for your situation. You should consult with a professional when appropriate. Neither the publisher nor the author shall be liable for any loss of profit or any other commercial damages, including but not limited to special, incidental, consequential, personal, or other damages.

Book Cover by Elena Chua

Medical Disclaimer

This book is intended to provide general health and wellness information and is not intended as a substitute for professional medical advice, diagnosis, or treatment. The author and publisher have made every effort to ensure that the information contained in this book is accurate and up-to-date. However, the medical field is continually evolving, and the readers are encouraged to consult a healthcare professional for any health concerns or before making any changes to their healthcare regimen.

The author and publisher expressly disclaim responsibility for any adverse effects arising from the use or application of the information contained in this book. No part of this book should be interpreted as a form of medical consultation or as a definitive guide to any specific treatment plan. Individual health concerns vary, and the advice and content provided in this book may not be suitable for everyone.

Readers should always seek the advice of their physician or other qualified health providers with any questions they may have regarding a medical condition or treatment options. Never disregard professional medical advice or delay seeking it because of something you have read in this book.

Contents

Introduction

In the intricate voyage of existence, pivotal transitions often go unrecognized—events that signify profound change. Menopause stands as one such event, historically misinterpreted and overshadowed by myths. Many women anticipate this phase with apprehension, viewing it as a farewell to their youthful essence. However, it's worth reevaluating this perspective. Could menopause be perceived not as a closure but as an invigorating commencement?

As a practitioner in the realm of medical aesthetics, I've been honored to guide numerous women through their menopausal transitions. I've observed their challenges, their victories, and their metamorphoses. These insights, grounded in genuine clinical interactions, are the core of this book. Being a woman, this is a path I am navigating too.

This book is not just about menopause; it's about embracing this remarkable phase of life with open arms. It's about understanding the power and potential that lie within it. It's about recognizing menopause is not the closing chapter of a woman's life, but the beginning of an exciting new one.

In these pages, we will embark on a journey of discovery—a journey that will unravel the mysteries of menopause, explore the changes it brings to your body and mind, and offer practical guidance on how to navigate this transformation with grace and confidence.

But this journey is more than just a scientific exploration. It's a celebration of womanhood and a testament to the strength and resilience of every woman who has ever faced this transition. It's a reminder that age is not a limitation, but a badge of honour—a symbol of wisdom, experience, and self-assuredness.

As we delve into the pages ahead, we will explore the physical and emotional changes that menopause can bring, busting myths along the way. We will delve into the realms of nutrition, exercise, and mental wellness, offering you the tools you need to not only survive but thrive during this life-altering phase.

But beyond the practical advice, we will uncover the stories of real women who have embarked on their own menopausal journeys, women who have emerged from this transformation stronger, wiser, and more vibrant than ever before. Their experiences serve as testaments to the potential that menopause holds—to shed the burdens of youth and embrace a newfound sense of self.

So, I invite you to turn the page and embark on this enlightening journey with an open heart and an eager spirit. Together, we will redefine menopause as not a conclusion, but a glorious commencement—a new beginning filled with endless possibilities, wisdom, and, above all, empowerment.

Chapter One

Debunking Menopausal Myths Through the Ages

Menopause is a word that carries with it a myriad of misconceptions and stereotypes. For far too long, society has painted a bleak picture of this natural life transition, casting it as a time of decline and despair. But, as we embark on this journey together, we must confront these myths head-on and discover the hidden truths beneath the surface.

One of the most pervasive myths surrounding menopause is the notion that it marks the end of a woman's relevance, beauty, and vitality. Nothing could be further from the truth. Menopause is not a full stop; it's a comma in the sentence of life. It's a phase that brings change, but change does not equate to diminishment. It's a transformation that, when embraced, can lead to personal growth and empowerment beyond measure.

Another common misconception is that menopause is solely a physical event, focusing solely on hot flashes and hormonal fluctuations. While these are part of the journey, they are not the entirety of it. Menopause encompasses emotional, psychological, and spiritual dimensions that deserve our attention. It's a time when you can tap into your inner strength, wisdom, and resilience, forging a deeper connection with your true self.

It's crucial to challenge the stereotype that menopause is a solitary path laden with suffering. In reality, countless women around the world are navigating this journey simultaneously. Sharing experiences, stories, and support can be an empowering part of the process.

As we delve into the fascinating world of menopause, it's crucial to confront the myths and misconceptions that have shrouded this natural life stage throughout history. These myths, often rooted in misunderstanding and cultural biases, have perpetuated stereotypes about menopausal women. By debunking these myths, we can pave the way for a more enlightened and empowering perspective on menopause. Let's look at some myths that surround women and menopause since the beginning of time.

The "Witching Hour" Myth

In mediaeval Europe, between the 15th and 18th centuries, a dark and sinister belief persisted – that menopausal women were associated with witchcraft. Their hormonal changes and mood swings were woefully misunderstood, leading to the unjust belief that they were possessed by evil spirits or capable of casting malevolent spells. This myth, fueled by ignorance, contributed to the persecution of countless women during the infamous witch trials.

Loss of Fertility Equals Worthlessness

Throughout history, across various cultures and time periods, women's worth was often inextricably linked to their ability to bear children. Menopause, marking the end of fertility, was tragically perceived as the end of a woman's value. Women who couldn't conceive were marginalised, their societal importance diminished. This pervasive myth has roots in societies worldwide, perpetuating the idea that a woman's worth extends far beyond her reproductive capabilities.

Menopause as a Disease

In the 19th century, particularly in Western countries, menopause was frequently treated as a medical ailment rather than a natural life transition. Physicians diagnosed women with "female hysteria" or "neurasthenia" and prescribed treatments like rest cures, electrical stimulation, or even hysterectomies to alleviate menopausal symptoms. This medicalization perpetuated the idea that menopause was a problem to be fixed rather than embraced.

The "Cold and Frigid" Stereotype

Throughout history, across cultures, a pervasive stereotype portrayed menopausal women as emotionally cold, unfeeling, or uninterested in intimacy. This oversimplified and misguided belief disregarded the emotional and sexual vitality that many women experience during and after menopause.

The "Crazy Cat Lady" Myth (20th Century, Western Countries)

In the 20th century, particularly in Western countries, an eccentric stereotype emerged, depicting menopausal women as obsessed with cats. This myth likely originated from a misunderstanding of the emotional changes associated with menopause. In reality, menopause can bring about a range of emotions, but it certainly doesn't turn women into cat enthusiasts.

Menopause as a Western Phenomenon (Various Cultures, Pre-Modern Times)

In some cultures, menopause was not widely recognized as a distinct life stage until more recent times. It was often overshadowed by other life events or simply not openly discussed. This lack of acknowledgement led to a dearth of support for women experiencing menopausal symptoms, irrespective of their cultural background.

By acknowledging these historical myths and misconceptions about menopause, we can appreciate how far we've come in our understanding of this transformative phase in a woman's life. As we embark on this journey together, let's continue to challenge stereotypes and embrace menopause as a time of personal growth, renewal, and empowerment.

In the chapters ahead, we'll explore how embracing menopause as a time of personal growth and empowerment can lead to a life filled with renewed purpose and passion. Together, we'll shatter the stereotypes, rewrite the narrative, and pave the way for a brighter, more empowered menopausal journey.

Chapter Two

Menopause Through History

Let's take a captivating journey through the annals of history to unravel the intriguing story of how menopause has been perceived, misunderstood, and ultimately liberated over the centuries. Prepare for a tour de force in historical hilarity and enlightening anecdotes.

Menopause in Ancient Times: Wisdom from the Ancients

In the distant past, menopause was seen as a passage to wisdom and grace. In Ancient Egypt, the Ebers Papyrus contained remedies for menopausal symptoms, including potions made from juniper berries and honey. The wisdom of the ancients celebrated this transition as a time when women could focus on guiding the next generation, though we must admit, honey potions might not have been the most effective treatment.

From Stigmatization to Suppression

Fast forward to the Middle Ages, a period where women's health took a nosedive. Menopause became the Voldemort of the medical world—nobody dared speak its name. Mediaeval physicians often prescribed herbs like black cohosh and chasteberry, but the effectiveness remained questionable. It's safe to say that these remedies didn't win any "Best Medicinal Elixir" awards.

The Era of Hysteria

The Victorian era brought us not only corsets and tea parties but also a curious diagnosis—hysteria. Women were diagnosed with hysteria for displaying symptoms like mood swings and hot flashes. The treatment? A visit to the doctor for a "hysterical paroxysm," which was basically a precursor to what we now know as vibrators. Yes, you read that right—the first vibrators were invented as a medical device to treat "hysteria." Talk about a shocking medical history!

From Suffrage to Healthcare

The late 19th and early 20th centuries marked a turning point for women's health. Suffragettes, like Susan B. Anthony and Elizabeth Cady Stanton, fought for women's rights, including control over their own bodies. Enter the indomitable Dr. Elizabeth Blackwell, the first woman to receive a medical degree in the United States. She shattered glass ceilings while helping women understand that menopause was just another part of life, not a curse to be endured.

A Contemporary Shift

Today, we're witnessing a seismic shift in understanding menopause. Women are taking control of their health decisions, armed with knowledge and confidence. The era of empowerment has dawned, and it's high time we bid adieu to the days of corsets and hysterics. With accurate information and a dash of humour, we're embracing menopause as a new beginning—a time of wisdom, strength, and yes, a few hot flashes along the way.

As we journey through history, we'll unveil the challenges women faced and the humorous anecdotes that peppered their struggles. From honey potions to "hysterical paroxysms," menopause's historical legacy is nothing short of astonishing. Together, we'll liberate women's health from the shackles of misunderstanding, paving the way for a brighter and more enlightened future.

Chapter Three

Navigating the Seasons of Change

This journey is all about reimagining perimenopause and menopause, shedding light on these transformative phases of a woman's life, and equipping you with the knowledge and tools to navigate them effectively. Whether you're experiencing symptoms in your mid-30s, 40s, 45s, or beyond, or you simply want to understand what lies ahead, you're in the right place.

As we embark on this journey together, let's delve into my patient Brenda's telling experiences with perimenopause. She, too, felt ill-prepared for the profound changes that accompanied this phase of life. At 55, she is still menstruating, even though the average age for menopause hovers around 51 to 52. However, her symptoms began much earlier, around the age of 35. Her menstrual cycle started to shift, coming closer together, and premenstrual syndrome became a regular companion. Emotionally, she felt overwhelmed, struggling to cope with the challenges of motherhood.

It was during this period that she sought help from her doctor, only to receive recommendations that didn't resonate with her. The standard advice of more exercise, less food, and possibly an antidepressant didn't feel right. Driven by her own experiences and her desire to help patients facing similar struggles, she embarked on a mission to unravel the mysteries of perimenopause and menopause.

As Brenda progressed through her 40s, 45s, and 50s, her symptoms evolved. Her menstrual cycles became even shorter, and she began experiencing night sweats and blood sugar issues. Alarmed by these changes, she started to investigate the hormonal intricacies of this phase of life, not just for herself but also for the countless women who were grappling with a lack of answers from conventional healthcare.

At the age of 35, Brenda's symptoms began to emerge. Her menstrual cycles, which had been a reliable 28-day affair, started creeping closer together—24 days, 25 days, 26 days. Alongside these physical changes, she grappled with heightened premenstrual syndrome (PMS). Emotionally, she felt like she was drowning, struggling to navigate the complexities of life. As a working mother, her days often stretched to 10 hours at the office, leaving her drained. The simple act of arriving home felt like preparing for a daunting task, as she summoned the strength to show up for her husband and baby. It was an inner battle—a sense of grappling in the darkness.

Seeking answers, she turned to her family doctor, hoping for guidance. Brenda poured out her concerns about her irregular periods, escalating stress levels, and the added challenge of weight management. Unfortunately, her doctor's response was underwhelming. The suggestions offered were to exercise more, eat less, and contemplate an antidepressant—a solution that didn't resonate with her. Deep inside, she knew there had to be more to her symptoms than simple prescriptions for a pill and lifestyle changes that felt inadequate.

This moment marked the genesis of her quest to unravel the intricate web of hormones in perimenopause and menopause. Our mission wasn't solely about preparing ourselves for the journey; it was also a passionate endeavour to assist other women navigating the same rocky terrain without guidance from their primary care physicians.

As Brenda ventured deeper into her 40s, followed by her 45s and 50s, her symptoms took on new forms. Her menstrual cycles continued to shrink, sometimes as close as 21 or 22 days apart. The week preceding her period brought night sweats and troubling fluctuations in her blood sugar levels. Alarmingly, her medical providers seemed nonchalant about these issues. Her fasting glucose levels continued to rise year after year, a trend that raised red flags for her. However, the medical establishment remained unresponsive.

It was around the age of 50 that memory issues began to surface. The sharpness of her mind, once akin to a steel trap, dulled, and the ability to recall every word in a sentence started to slip through her fingers. Her cognitive functions seemed to require a bit more effort, a subtle but unsettling shift.

If any of these experiences resonate with you, rest assured, you are not alone, and you are in precisely the right place. Our journey through this book aims to shine a light on the intricate biological mechanisms at play. Understanding these mechanisms will empower you to seek out solutions that align seamlessly with your body's natural rhythms, providing lasting relief and restored harmony.

Embracing the Perimenopause and Menopause Journey

Perimenopause and menopause are much more than just biological events—they're profound initiations into a new phase of life. This is your opportunity to step back from the dominant culture's expectations and take a closer look at your life. It's a time for introspection and self-discovery: Are you living life on your own terms, or are you still following the scripts written by your parents or society?

Perimenopause, often referred to as the period around menopause, is a unique journey that can span a few months to several decades, depending on how attuned you are to its symptoms. Behind the scenes, significant changes are taking place in your body. If you still have your ovaries, they begin producing fewer and fewer sex hormones, starting with progesterone, followed by oestrogen, and sometimes even testosterone for some of us. As hormone levels drop below a certain threshold, perimenopausal symptoms can begin to emerge.

These symptoms can manifest in various ways—physically and emotionally. You might experience breast tenderness, notice the growth of fibroids in your uterus, or have heavier menstrual bleeding. Emotionally, you might find yourself more irritable, struggling with heightened premenstrual syndrome, or even facing premenstrual dysphoric disorder (PMDD). Keep in mind that the symptoms can vary significantly from one woman to another.

Menopause, on the other hand, is defined as the absence of a menstrual period for a full year. It's a biological milestone, a day that marks your one-year anniversary since your last period. In many ways, menopause is a celebration, an acknowledgement of this transformative phase. You might even consider throwing yourself a menopause party to honour this momentous occasion.

However, menopause is not just a biological construct; it's also a socio-cultural one. Society often places an overwhelming emphasis on youth culture, causing many women to feel like they are gradually fading into the background as they enter menopause. This societal narrative can make women feel sidelined or dismissed, which can be disheartening.

It's essential to challenge this narrative and recognise the value and wisdom that women bring during perimenopause and menopause. This phase is an opportunity for self-discovery, self-care, and self-appreciation. It's a time when women can come together to support each other, activating the power of oxytocin and oestrogen to foster deep bonds, connections, love, and support.

By embracing perimenopause and menopause as an initiation into a new phase of life, women can rewrite the script and reclaim their place in society. It's about celebrating the wisdom and experiences that come with age, finding strength in unity, and emerging from this journey with newfound confidence and self-awareness.

Navigating the Landscape of Perimenopause

Perimenopause is a remarkable phase of a woman's life, and it's often accompanied by a significant transformation in perspective. During our reproductive years, which span from puberty until we start cycling less predictably, typically around ages 35 to 45, we operate under the influence of varying levels of oestrogen, progesterone, and testosterone throughout our menstrual cycle. These hormonal fluctuations compel us to adapt, accommodate, and sometimes even tolerate circumstances, almost like a rehearsal for people-pleasers.

However, when perimenopause arrives, and the predictable daily hormonal regimen begins to wane, something truly remarkable happens. The hormonal veil lifts, and we find ourselves speaking our truth, perhaps for the very first time. This is what excites me most about perimenopause and menopause—the opportunity it offers to step into our power, make deliberate choices about our lives, and examine behaviours like people-pleasing to discern whether they continue to serve us. Understanding our bodies and hormones empowers us to speak our truth authentically and embark on a profound initiation process.

Now, let's delve into what perimenopause and menopause are and how oestrogen takes centre stage in this transition.

Oestrogen is undeniably the leading character in the middle-life transformation that women undergo. It acts as a primary regulator of the female body, playing various roles at different stages of life. At birth, oestrogen levels are minimal, but they begin to fluctuate significantly during puberty. This hormonal shift brings forth various changes, such as acne, breast development, and menstruation, marking a critical phase of female development.

During your reproductive years, typically your 20s, 30s, and sometimes into your 40s, oestrogen levels stabilise—however, perimenopause ushers in a transformation akin to puberty in reverse. Initially, progesterone levels begin to decline, while oestrogen fluctuates wildly. Subsequently, oestrogen levels follow suit, declining further during menopause. At this stage, oestrogen, progesterone, and even testosterone may reach low levels, giving rise to a myriad of symptoms.

Perimenopause is the period around menopause, lasting approximately a decade, typically from ages 42 to 52. It's during this time that women experience subtle yet impactful changes. These changes often begin with alterations in the menstrual cycle but can expand to encompass emotional symptoms such as irritability, mood swings, depression, and even physical manifestations like hot flashes, night sweats, changes in sex drive, joint stiffness, and more. All these symptoms are intricately connected to the shifts in oestrogen, progesterone, and testosterone levels.

To identify if you're in perimenopause, you may encounter some common signs and questions. For instance, you might feel a diminished enthusiasm for household responsibilities or experience social withdrawal, preferring solitude over social gatherings. Weight gain, especially around the abdomen, may become noticeable due to shifts in insulin sensitivity caused by hormonal changes. Emotional instability, with amplified emotions, might take centre stage. Exercise may lose its appeal, and you may find it challenging to maintain a fitness routine. Sleep disturbances, including waking up in the middle of the night, can disrupt your rest. Changes in grooming habits, decreased interest in personal appearance, and an increase in wrinkles may become evident.

Furthermore, perimenopause can lead to unpredictable menstrual cycles, ranging from heavy to light flow, spotting to heavy bleeding, and irregular timing. Additionally, you may find yourself craving chocolate or alcohol more than desire sexual intimacy. These manifestations encompass the complex landscape of perimenopause, which can be both challenging and transformative.

Understanding these nuances is essential for embracing this transition with grace and empowerment.

Unpacking the Impact of Hormones on Your Sex Drive and Lifestyle

Sex drive, a powerful and innate aspect of our human experience, often takes centre stage in conversations about perimenopause and menopause. It's worth noting that around 70% of your sex drive is influenced by hormones, making them pivotal players in this intricate story. The hormonal changes accompanying perimenopause and menopause can indeed put a damper on your libido.

However, there's more to this tale. As women navigate the terrain of perimenopause and menopause, they often find themselves grappling with the prospect of making significant lifestyle changes to not only survive but thrive during this transition. These changes may include bidding farewell to sugar, and processed foods, embracing regular exercise, lifting heavy weights, and incorporating meditation into their daily routines. Yet, these adjustments can seem daunting, even overwhelming, causing some to question how to fit them into their lives. Interestingly, this hesitance to embrace behaviour change is, in itself, a symptom of perimenopause. It's essential to recognise that if you're feeling less enthusiastic about making these shifts, you're not alone, and there's good news—we have practical solutions that can be implemented gradually, allowing you to make progress at your own pace. These small steps can eventually lead to remarkable transformations.

We've delved into the starring roles of oestrogen, progesterone, and testosterone in the perimenopausal journey. However, it's crucial to remember that hormones don't operate in isolation. They function within a complex hormonal symphony, and three other hormones demand our attention—oestrogen, cortisol, and thyroid.

Oestrogen, as we've discussed, holds the primary regulator position in the female body. It shares an intricate dance with progesterone, akin to Tango partners. Achieving balance between these two hormones is vital, as neither should dominate the other. But oestrogen doesn't stop there; it also engages in a significant crosstalk with thyroid hormones. The thyroid is like the gas pedal of your metabolism, influencing the rate you burn calories and impacting various cellular processes.

However, the star of the show, in some respects, is cortisol. Often described as the highest-priority hormone, cortisol plays an indispensable role. It regulates your blood sugar levels, orchestrates your stress response (fight, flight, freeze), and modulates your immune system. Without cortisol, your body would face profound challenges.

Therefore, while oestrogen, progesterone, and testosterone understandably garner attention, we must recognise the broader orchestra that includes oestrogen, cortisol, and thyroid. These hormones work in harmony to support your well-being. However, when their synergy is disrupted, it can trigger the symptoms you might encounter during perimenopause and menopause.

Understanding the Symptoms of Menopause

In our journey through perimenopause and menopause, understanding the intricate hormonal changes is essential. The average age for menopause is around 51 to 52 years old. The range of symptoms associated with perimenopause encompasses weight gain, fibroids, increased cramping, breast tenderness, irritability, heightened hunger, insomnia, vaginal dryness, loss of libido, and more. As perimenopause progresses into menopause, additional symptoms emerge, such as hot flashes, night sweats, breast cancer concerns, depression, heart disease, increased vaginal discomfort, osteoporosis, and incontinence.

What's crucial to grasp here is that many of these symptoms, particularly mood swings, hot flashes, night sweats, low libido, and insomnia, are not solely attributable to ovarian changes. Instead, they originate in the female brain. It's a common misconception to view perimenopause and menopause as solely ovarian events, but the truth is that profound alterations occur in the female brain, playing a pivotal role in driving these symptoms.

In functional medicine, we adopt a systems-thinking approach, recognising that your body operates as an intricate system, with each component influencing the others. So, as we delve deeper into this journey, keep in mind that understanding these brain-driven changes is a key aspect of navigating perimenopause and menopause successfully.

A Dive into the Systems Biology of Perimenopause and Menopause

To fully grasp the complexities of perimenopause and menopause, let's embark on a brief science journey into the systems biology that governs these transitions.

Your body operates like a well-oiled machine in your pre-menopausal years, especially if you have regular 28 to 30-day menstrual cycles. During this time, your body experiences a daily ebb and flow of hormones, with testosterone peaking around day 14, oestrogen reaching its pinnacle around day 12, and progesterone hitting its peak at around day 21 or 22. These hormone fluctuations form the norm for your body's hormonal symphony.

However, as you approach the age range of 35 to 45, the system begins to show signs of strain. Imagine your body's control centre, the hypothalamus and pituitary in the brain, as the boss of your endocrine orchestra. They oversee your ovaries and your thyroid and adrenal glands, which are responsible for producing crucial hormones like cortisol, pregnenolone, and DHEA. It's a tightly regulated dance that ensures hormonal harmony.

But, as you start to exhaust your ovarian egg supply, this once precise feedback loop between your brain and ovaries starts to falter. The hypothalamus and pituitary, your hormonal conductors, begin to lose their grip. This shift typically occurs sometime between the ages of 35 and 45.

Moreover, for those who have experienced significant trauma, be it during childhood or adulthood, this can disrupt your body's stress response system and, consequently, the hormonal control system. Such individuals often face a more challenging perimenopausal and menopausal journey with rockier symptoms.

So, we must consider the triad of oestrogen, progesterone, and testosterone and the intricate interplay between oestrogen, cortisol, and thyroid. Understanding how this control system can sometimes malfunction before entering perimenopause is crucial, as it can significantly impact your transition.

Many women wonder whether hormone testing can provide insights into their hormonal status. The answer is yes. If your healthcare provider dismisses the idea due to hormone fluctuations, I encourage you to seek a more collaborative clinician. Hormone tests offer valuable information throughout perimenopause and menopause.

During the first phase of perimenopause, when progesterone starts to dwindle, you can check your progesterone levels, usually on day 21 or 22, to assess if they're 10 or higher. A level below that indicates diminishing progesterone and may result in shorter menstrual cycles, increased anxiety and disrupted sleep.

In the second half of perimenopause, as oestrogen also declines, you'll observe that your estradiol levels no longer peak around day 12. Measuring estradiol can help determine whether you're in phase one or phase two of perimenopause.

Hormone therapy during perimenopause typically focuses on supplementing what's missing. In the initial phase, when progesterone is low, natural progesterone may be prescribed, especially for those battling sleep issues. In the latter phase, where both progesterone and oestrogen levels drop, treatment often entails both hormones, provided the patient is a suitable candidate.

Navigating Hormone Therapy and Tackling Weight Gain

In the first half of perimenopause, when progesterone levels drop, and you find your menstrual cycles becoming closer together, sleep disruptions, and heightened anxiety, progesterone therapy can offer significant relief. However, it's crucial to note that I recommend progesterone therapy solely during perimenopause, not in menopause.

Moving on to the second half of perimenopause and into menopause, when symptoms like memory issues, vaginal dryness, mood changes, and other signs of low oestrogen emerge, I often recommend combining oestrogen and progesterone therapy. This combination provides the necessary support to alleviate these symptoms and is suitable for this later phase of perimenopause as well as menopause.

Now, let's address the common concern of weight gain during this life transition. It's not uncommon to experience a metabolic crisis, which typically sets in after the age of 40, although some may notice it earlier. You might find yourself struggling to shed excess weight, regardless of your efforts.

This weight gain is linked to changes beneath the surface, mainly how oestrogen and insulin interact within your body. Oestrogen levels decline, and with less soothing progesterone, sleep quality can diminish, leading to elevated cortisol levels. This hormonal upheaval contributes to a shift in fat distribution, with less fat accumulating in the breast and hip areas and more around the belly—a frustrating phenomenon many of us encounter.

Additionally, a shift occurs in the relationship between insulin and oestrogen. After reaching their 40s, women tend to gain approximately five pounds of fat and lose about five pounds of muscle every decade. This process can continue unless specific measures are taken to address insulin levels and ensure a healthy metabolic state.

To mitigate weight gain during this transition, paying close attention to your diet is essential. Your food choices significantly impact your hormonal balance and insulin regulation. Monitoring your insulin levels and striving for metabolic flexibility, where your body can efficiently utilise both carbohydrates and ketones, is crucial. In the following chapters, you will read about what has worked for my patients– the ketogenic diet and fasting.

Metabolic Health Check: Understanding Glucose, HbA1C, and Insulin in the Menopausal Journey

Regularly monitoring fasting glucose, haemoglobin A1c levels (HbA1C), and fasting insulin is a proactive approach to safeguarding metabolic health. As women traverse the menopausal transition, managing insulin and properly nourishing hormones become pivotal in countering the notorious weight gain often associated with this phase of life.

A brief look at fasting glucose reveals its utility: gauging the concentration of glucose in the blood after an overnight fast. This snapshot illuminates the body's proficiency in regulating glucose devoid of recent food intake. When these levels rise, it may foreshadow impaired glucose regulation, a doorway to type 2 diabetes.

Delving into HbA1c, or glycated haemoglobin, unveils its unique makeup. Chemically bonded with glucose, HbA1c serves as a temporal marker, reflecting average blood glucose over 2 to 3 months. Given the 120-day lifespan of red blood cells, HbA1c levels intimate the glucose exposure these cells have encountered. Elevated levels point towards a protracted phase of heightened blood glucose, signalling potential glucose regulation issues. Beyond diagnosis, HbA1c plays a pivotal role in tracking diabetes progression.

Fasting insulin directly from the pancreas mirrors the insulin count after an overnight fast. Its primary function? Facilitating glucose absorption from the bloodstream to the cells. By gauging fasting insulin, one can discern potential insulin resistance, a scenario where the body's cells resist insulin's overtures. The aftermath? Escalated insulin production to stabilise blood glucose. Early detection of heightened fasting insulin can forewarn against impending insulin resistance, a precursor to metabolic syndrome, type 2 diabetes, heart ailments, and associated metabolic disorders.

This becomes an accentuated concern for women, especially during the menopause corridor. The hormonal tide during menopause can recalibrate insulin sensitivity, escalating the risk matrix for type 2 diabetes. Add to this the propensity for midlife weight gain, tethered to these hormonal oscillations, and the urgency for metabolic health monitoring becomes clear. In sum, for those either approaching or navigating menopause, these metrics crystallise into an essential toolkit, spotlighting the nuances of metabolic health impacted by hormonal shifts.

This marks the end of our quick journey through the menopause landscape, and you might be thinking, "That's a lot of information to absorb." Rest assured, as we progress through the book, we'll delve deeper into these details, providing you with a comprehensive understanding of the solutions you can implement step by step.

Chapter Four

Dissecting the Saturated Fat Paradox

Have you ever questioned why men and women accumulate fat in different patterns and locations? Why is it that during puberty, boys often gain muscle while girls experience fat gain in specific areas like the hips, buttocks, and breasts? And what about the phenomenon of women gaining weight as they approach menopause? These questions lead us to a fascinating exploration of the intricate relationship between gender, hormones, and fat distribution.

One of the key factors we must understand about menopause is the gradual reduction of oestrogen in a woman's body. Strangely, as oestrogen levels decline, the risk of coronary artery narrowing increases. This is a notable shift from the protective role that oestrogen used to play in guarding the artery walls and preventing the buildup of plaque.

Now, let's confront the saturated fat myth: the belief that saturated fat is a major contributor to heart disease, and consequently, adhering to a low-fat diet can mitigate this risk. This idea has been deeply ingrained in medical education for decades, leading many, including myself, down the path of limited fat intake and, in some cases, vegetarianism. However, it's time to challenge this long-standing premise.

Redefining the Fat Story: French Paradox and Inuit Insights

Consider the "French paradox," a puzzling observation where the French maintain low rates of coronary heart disease (CHD) deaths despite their high consumption of dietary cholesterol and saturated fat. This concept emerged in the 1980s, challenging the established norms.

Traditional Inuit diets provide another intriguing case study. Inuit populations derive about 50% of their calories from fat, with minimal carbohydrates, primarily glycogen from raw meat. Despite their high intake of saturated fat and low carbohydrate consumption, they exhibit low rates of heart disease, seemingly contradicting the prevailing belief linking saturated fat to heart problems.

Heart Myths Busted: Fat, Facts, and the Saturated Story

As we continue our journey, let's explore the evidence that contradicts the notion that saturated fat is a leading cause of heart disease:

In 2009, an expert consultation by the Food & Agriculture Organization at the WHO found that available evidence from cohort and randomised controlled trials was unsatisfactory and unreliable for making judgments about the effects of dietary fat on CHD.

A 2010 meta-analysis of prospective epidemiologic studies published in the American Journal of Clinical Nutrition failed to provide significant evidence linking dietary saturated fat to an increased risk of CHD or cardiovascular disease (CVD).

In a comprehensive 2014 meta-analysis led by Rajiv Chowdhury and his team, the association between different fatty acids and the risk of coronary disease was meticulously explored. This analysis synthesised data from many observational studies and randomised controlled trials, encompassing several hundreds of thousands of participants. The results were enlightening: comparing the highest and lowest dietary fatty acid intakes revealed no definitive correlation between saturated, monounsaturated, or the majority of polyunsaturated fatty acids and elevated coronary risk. This research casts doubt on the current cardiovascular guidelines, which strongly favour consuming polyunsaturated fatty acids while advising against saturated fats. Echoing this sentiment, the authors explicitly stated, "The prevailing evidence did not firmly support cardiovascular guidelines that encouraged high consumption of polyunsaturated fats (PUFA) and low consumption of saturated fats."

These findings challenge the conventional narrative. However, let's also consider historical studies that have shaped our understanding of dietary fat and heart disease.

The Framingham Heart Study in the 1940s initially suggested a positive link between cholesterol and heart disease. However, further investigation revealed that cholesterol had no predictive value for heart disease in women above 50. Moreover, when the men's diets with high versus low cholesterol were examined, there was no association between the amount or type of fat consumed and heart disease.

In 1957, a study involving 5,400 male employees of the Western Electric Company over 4.5 years found no significant difference in coronary-related mortality rates between those with high-fat diets and those with leaner diets. A follow-up study in 1981 reaffirmed these findings.

One of the most notable moments in the discourse surrounding saturated fats emerged from the 1973 Minnesota Coronary Experiment (MCE). This expansive study unfolded in a nursing home and six state mental hospitals in Minnesota, USA, involving a vast participant group of 9,423 individuals aged between 20 and 97. The dietary regimen for the intervention group was tailored to replace saturated fats, often sourced from animal fats, standard margarine, and shortenings, with linoleic acid, predominantly from corn oil and polyunsaturated margarine. The participants were categorised into two groups based on their diets: a high-fat diet (18%) and a low-fat diet (9%). What was startling was that there was no discernible difference in heart disease occurrences or mortality rates between the two factions. However, the real shocker was the concealment of these findings, which remained in the shadows for 16 years.

Fast forward to 2016, when scholars revisited this long-forgotten data from the MCE, held between 1968 and 1973. The core aim was to evaluate if trading saturated fat for linoleic acid-rich vegetable oil could curtail the onset of coronary heart disease and death by slashing serum cholesterol levels. Though the study found that the intervention group did exhibit a marked decrease in serum cholesterol levels compared to the control group (a significant drop of 13.8% against a mere 1.0% from their initial levels), there was no evident mortality benefit. More worryingly, for every 30 mg/dL dip in serum cholesterol, there was a 22% spike in the risk of death. Additionally, the initiative showed no apparent advantages concerning coronary atherosclerosis or myocardial infarcts.

Zooming out further, a systematic review that brought together data from five other randomised controlled trials, incorporating

10,808 participants, mirrored the objectives of the MCE. The goal? Lowering cholesterol through diet. Yet again, the findings were sobering. The overarching conclusion from these collective efforts was that while substituting saturated fat with linoleic acid brought down serum cholesterol levels, the projected health benefits, notably a reduced mortality risk from coronary heart disease or other causes, were absent. This revelation from the MCE underscores a distressing trend in scientific inquiries — the withholding or selective publication of results, which can inadvertently paint a rosier picture of specific dietary shifts, like transitioning from saturated fats to linoleic acid-infused vegetable oils.

In 1977, an NIH cohort study made a noteworthy discovery. It found that high LDL cholesterol was only a marginal risk factor for heart disease, primarily for individuals over 50. A better predictor of heart disease was low HDL cholesterol levels, and high triglycerides were equally strong indicators. The study suggested that factors raising HDL should be considered for reducing CHD risk.

Fast forward to 2001, when the Cochrane Collaboration conducted a meta-analysis of 27 randomised controlled trials involving over 10,000 subjects, each followed for an average of 3 years. The analysis found that saturated fat did not impact longevity or cardiovascular events. In 2006, a follow-up meta-analysis by the Cochrane Collaboration indicated that multiple risk factor interventions did not affect mortality for preventing CHD.

The 1990s bore witness to the dominance of the low-fat, high-starch diet heralded by the USDA food guide pyramid. However, a surge of evidence indicated its inefficacy for weight loss, heart disease, and specific cancer prevention. A critical assessment came from an eight-year study involving nearly 49,000 women: the Women's Health Initiative Dietary Modification Trial. This trial, initiated in 1993, was driven by the perception of dietary fat as harmful. With substantial funding, researchers roped in women aged between 50 to 79. Aiming to reduce fat intake from 38% to 20% of their diet, 19,541 participants were advised to embrace a low-fat diet.

Meanwhile, another 29,294 women continued their regular diets. However, after eight years, outcomes revealed no significant benefits of the low-fat diet in reducing risks of breast cancer, colorectal cancer, or cardiovascular disease. Even more shocking was the discovery that for every 30 mg/dL reduction in serum cholesterol, there was a 22% rise in mortality risk.

The Women's Health Initiative Dietary Modification Trial's findings were unexpected to many, as the low-fat narrative had been pervasive for years. Yet, extended studies, such as the Nurses Health Study, have consistently shown negligible connections between fat calorie percentage and risks of major diseases like breast cancer or heart disease. Recent comprehensive reviews have shifted the focus from low fat intake to the nature of the fat consumed.

The Saturated Fat Scapegoat and the Sugar Industry's Influence

Have you ever wondered how saturated fat became the villain in the narrative of coronary heart disease? In the 1960s, a strategic move by the sugar industry came to light. Documents uncovered reveal that the industry had paid scientists to shift the blame for heart disease away from sugar, highlighting saturated fat as the primary cause instead. This influential payment, as shown by the documents unearthed by a researcher at the University of California, San Francisco, was published in the JAMA Internal Medicine journal in 2016. These findings point to a concerning trend suggesting that many dietary recommendations and related research spanning five decades may have been shaped, or even skewed, under the influence of the sugar industry's funding and preferences.

This intrigue began with the Sugar Research Foundation, presently known as the Sugar Association. They provided financial incentives, equating to about $50,000 in today's money, to three Harvard scientists. The aim? To produce a 1967 review in the prominent New England Journal of Medicine. This review, curated with research handpicked by the sugar group, effectively downplayed the health risks associated with sugar. In contrast, it placed significant emphasis on the dangers of saturated fat.

While this strategic play by the sugar industry was almost half a century ago, there is growing concern that such corporate influence on scientific research has never truly ceased. A notable example is a recent revelation in The New York Times where Coca-Cola, a giant in the sugary beverage industry, had been revealed to fund researchers generously. What is the primary objective of these researchers? To diminish the established link between sugary drinks and the obesity epidemic.

The unearthed documents also illuminate the intricacies of the debate regarding the adverse health implications of sugar as compared to saturated fat. Dr. Glantz, an author of the JAMA Internal Medicine paper, indicated the significance of such industry-funded reviews. When these are published in reputable journals, they profoundly shape the trajectory of the entire scientific discourse, often for decades.

What's even more alarming is the subsequent roles some of these paid scientists assumed. For instance, one of the beneficiaries of the sugar industry's funds, Dr. Mark Hegsted, later occupied a pivotal position as the head of nutrition at the U.S. Department of Agriculture. Here, he significantly contributed to the early federal dietary guidelines set out in 1977. These guidelines, while highlighting the health risks associated with saturated fats, merely described sugar as a contributor to tooth decay, vastly underplaying its other health implications.

This revelation serves as a resounding call to the scientific community and policymakers about the inherent risks and biases of industry-funded research. It underscores the pressing need for research to be underpinned by unbiased, public funding to ensure its integrity and credibility. The unveiling of this hidden truth serves as a stark reminder of the power of industry influence on scientific research and dietary recommendations. It also sheds light on how the narrative surrounding saturated fat took shape and influenced dietary guidelines, affecting the choices and health of millions.

The journey through these discoveries challenges long-held beliefs about dietary fat, heart disease, and menopause. It's a journey that underscores the complexity of these issues and the need for a nuanced, evidence-based approach to nutrition and health. As we navigate the intricate web of dietary myths and realities, we aim to arrive at a clearer understanding of how our choices impact our well-being, especially during pivotal life stages like menopause.

Decoding Cholesterol: Beyond the Numbers on Your Report

We now know that consuming cholesterol doesn't directly spike your blood cholesterol levels, as once believed. But when it comes to those cholesterol figures on your medical report, are you left scratching your head? Dive with me into the depths of these numbers to decode their significance. If you're not one for the nitty-gritty details, feel free to skim over. However, if understanding your health is on your radar, stay on board!

Cholesterol is essential. We can't live without it. While foods like eggs and meat contribute to our cholesterol, our body is a cholesterol factory on its own. The figures in your report reflect a mix of dietary intake and what your body produces.

Let's simplify: cholesterol primarily exists in two versions:

1. "Free" Cholesterol (UC): This type is easily used and stored by our body.

2. "Bound" Cholesterol (CE): Mostly what we get from food. Our body often finds it harder to use and tends to discard it.

Most cholesterol inside us isn't from that juicy steak we had last week; our body produces a good chunk of it!

Cholesterol isn't a great traveller on its own. Imagine trying to mix oil and water. To move around, our body packs cholesterol into tiny protein "suitcases" or lipoproteins. As these travel, they lighten their load, becoming more packed with cholesterol. Special proteins act as GPS for these "suitcases", guiding them efficiently throughout our body.

When you hear about "bad" cholesterol, you usually hear about LDL-C (that's usually the one on your blood test report). But there's more to the story:

- LDL-C: This measures the *amount* of bad cholesterol. Think of it as checking how much weight is in a suitcase.

- LDL-P: This measures the *number* of cholesterol "suitcases" (or lipoproteins). It's like counting how many suitcases you have.

Research shows that it's not just the weight in the suitcase (LDL-C) that's important, but the number of suitcases (LDL-P) matters even more. Why? Because having many tiny cholesterol-packed "suitcases" can be riskier for heart health than having a few heavier ones.

Surprisingly, some folks with perfect LDL-C levels (healthy amounts of bad cholesterol) still face heart risks because they have a high LDL-P (too many cholesterol "suitcases").

When cholesterol, especially the tiny suitcases (LDL-P), sticks to our arteries, blockages can form. This is the start of heart issues. It's a reminder that looking at both the amount (LDL-C) and the number (LDL-P) is crucial for understanding our heart risk.

Interpreting cholesterol tests can be as tricky as deciphering conflicting weather forecasts. One might predict sunshine, while another foresees a downpour. This is why it's crucial to consider both LDL-C and LDL-P when gauging heart health. Evaluating additional heart markers like HDL(high-density lipoprotein) and TG (triglycerides) further enriches our understanding, ensuring we don't hastily react to a single cholesterol reading. After all, cholesterol isn't just a mere line on a medical report – it's central to our overall well-being, especially our cardiovascular health. And for a comprehensive view, we must consider not just its volume but also the variety of its carriers in our body.

Chapter Five

Beyond Calorie Counting

Conventional advice for women approaching or experiencing menopause often revolves around adopting a low-fat, low-calorie diet. We have already shown that saturated fat does not cause heart disease, but does it increase the risk of obesity in a menopausal woman? This guidance is based on the notion that all calories are equal – the simplistic idea that it's all about "calories in versus calories out." However, delving deeper, we realise that not all calories are created equal. For instance, comparing 100 calories from rice to 100 calories from fat reveals vast differences in nutritional value and metabolic impact.

This view oversimplifies the complex issue of obesity and fails to explain why women tend to accumulate fat below the waist, while men often gain it above their waist. It doesn't clarify why boys undergo muscle gain during puberty while girls experience fat accumulation. Furthermore, it offers no insight into why women may gain weight during menopause even when their calorie intake and exercise habits remain unchanged.

Have you ever questioned the long-held belief that achieving a calorie deficit is the ultimate solution to weight loss? For centuries, physicians have advocated calorie-restricted diets as the remedy for weight loss, especially for women entering menopause, with limited success. Let's explore this myth and uncover the hidden complexities.

The Minnesota Starvation Experiment

In the early years of World War II, a pioneering study led by Ancel Keys at the University of Minnesota set out to investigate the effects of starvation on weight loss. Thirty-six conscientious objectors volunteered as test subjects, embarking on a gruelling journey. They endured 24 weeks of semi-starvation, consuming only 1600 calories per day—a regimen that today would be considered a healthy, low-fat diet. Their diet included whole wheat bread, cereal, ample servings of turnips and cabbage, and modest amounts of meat and dairy.

During the first 12 weeks, these men shed a pound of body fat per week, but their weight loss gradually slowed to just a quarter pound weekly in the following 12 weeks, despite ongoing deprivation. Over nearly half a year, they lost a mere 15 pounds of fat. However, this wasn't the only toll they paid. They constantly felt cold, their metabolism slowed, they experienced hair loss, their libidos waned, and they became preoccupied with thoughts of food day and night—symptoms now referred to as "semi-starvation neurosis." Four subjects even developed character neurosis, with two suffering breakdowns—one displayed weeping, suicidal thoughts, and violent outbursts, leading to hospitalisation. The others experienced personality deterioration that culminated in two separate attempts at self-mutilation—one subject nearly severed a fingertip with an axe, and when that failed to end the study, he accidentally chopped off three fingers.

The post-starvation observations were also eye-opening. Many, once reintroduced to regular food, reported insatiable hunger, consuming up to 5,000 calories daily. They rapidly regained weight, with many overshooting their initial weights. Within 20 weeks of recovery, they were, on average, 50% fatter than when they began—a phenomenon now known as "post-starvation obesity." Intriguingly, some developed body image issues, feeling "overweight" despite being undernourished. This rebound effect is now commonly termed "yo-yo dieting."

Furthermore, this restraint resulted in a reduction in energy expenditure, highlighting that calorie restriction alone is not the answer to controlling weight gain, especially during life stages like menopause. Ancel Keys concluded that a restrictive caloric intake not only jeopardises physical health but also severely impairs mental well-being. It wasn't about willpower; it was pure human physiology.

This painstaking study is one of the most meticulous investigations into the long-term effects of low-calorie, low-fat diets on the body and mind. In an ironic twist, today's diet culture still advocates for calorie-restrictive diets eerily reminiscent of the "starvation" phase in Keys' experiment. Diets recommending 1,500 or even 1,200 calories daily are commonplace, as evidenced by numerous diet books and guidelines.

Sumo's Secret: Carbs, Calories, and Colossal Size

Intriguingly, a visit to Nagoya, Japan, led to an unexpected revelation about extreme body weight and diets. Witnessing a sumo match, I couldn't help but wonder about the dietary habits of these enormous athletes. Sumo wrestlers in Japan typically reach weights exceeding 300 pounds by their early 20s. In 1976, researchers from the University of Tokyo, led by Sunae Mishizawa, published a comprehensive article in the American Journal of Clinical Nutrition—the most extensive literature on sumo diet, body composition, and health.

Professional sumo wrestling is divided into two groups: the upper group, consisting of the country's best wrestlers, and the lower group. The upper group consumes an average of 5500 calories daily, primarily from "chunko nabe" (pork stew), with 57% of their diet being carbohydrates and only 16% fat. Remarkably, this carb-rich, low-fat diet provides twice the carb intake of an average Japanese diet—a far cry from what public health guidelines in the United States would consider a feasible low-fat target.

On the other hand, the lower group of sumo wrestlers, despite achieving similar weights to their upper-group counterparts, exhibited higher body fat percentages and less muscle mass. They consumed approximately 5100 calories per day, with 87% of their diet being carbohydrates and 9% fat.

If one were to design a diet aimed at inducing pathological obesity, it might resemble this low-fat, high-carb regimen—a stark parallel to the dietary advice often given to postmenopausal women to reduce their risk of heart disease, albeit at a more moderate calorie intake. Notably, the high-carb content may play a pivotal role in allowing such extraordinary overconsumption, sustained not just for days but for years, even decades.

Carbs vs. Fats: Unveiling the Surprising Weight Loss Battle

In 2007, Christopher Gardner conducted a study involving 320 pre-menopausal women, aiming to uncover the impact of carbohydrates and fats on weight loss. The study embraced four popular diets, each representing a distinct dietary approach, and followed the women over 12 months. These diets ranged from the extreme:

- Atkins: Low carb, high fat

- Zone: Moderately carb-restricted

- Learn: USDA balanced diet

- Ornish: Low fat, high carb, notable for its exclusion of refined carbs and processed foods.

The study's format was straightforward: 311 premenopausal, overweight, and obese women were divided into groups, each following a distinct diet for 12 months. The Atkins, Zone, LEARN, and Ornish diets were all under the microscope. Christopher Gardner, a vegan himself and naturally sceptical, conducted the study. After 12 months, the results were illuminating.

Weight loss, the primary metric, saw Atkins (high fat, low carbohydrate diet) participants shedding an impressive average of 4.7 kg over the year. In comparison, the next best performer, the LEARN diet, trailed with an average loss of 2.6 kg. The Ornish and Zone diets lagged even further behind.

But the benefits of the Atkins diet didn't stop at mere weight loss. The study also meticulously recorded a range of metabolic markers — and once again, Atkins shone brightly. Participants in the Atkins group demonstrated significant reductions in triglycerides (TG) and increases in high-density lipoprotein (HDL), both critical risk factors for coronary heart disease (CHD). This suggests that not only were participants losing weight, but their overall metabolic health was experiencing a significant boost. It's a dual victory that few diets can claim.

These studies reveal a complex truth about weight loss and diets, challenging the conventional wisdom of calorie counting and shedding light on the role of carbohydrates and fats in managing weight, especially during life transitions like menopause. Christopher D Gardner's study offers more than just numbers; it provides a compelling testament to a high-fat, low-carbohydrate diet's robustness. It's not merely about shedding weight but embracing a holistic approach that enhances overall health and well-being.

Chapter Six

Unlocking the Hormonal Puzzle of Obesity

The Old Thought on Weight Gain

For a long time, many believed that gaining weight was all about eating too many calories and not burning enough off. This idea suggested that all calories impacted our body in the same way. So, to lose weight, the solution seemed simple - eat less and exercise more. However, this approach often fails in the long run. Why? Because reducing your food intake makes your body react in ways that fight weight loss.

The Body's Response to Caloric Reduction: A Double-Edged Sword

When one reduces their calorie intake, the body, in its innate wisdom, perceives this as a potential threat to survival. While the intention might be weight loss, the body interprets this sudden drop in energy supply as a sign of scarcity or impending famine. Consequently, it triggers several adaptive responses to conserve energy and ensure its survival.

Firstly, the metabolic rate slows down. This is the body's primary defence mechanism against starvation. A slower metabolism means the body burns fewer calories at rest, making weight loss more challenging than initially anticipated. Simultaneously, levels of the hunger hormone ghrelin increase. This can lead to heightened feelings of hunger, making reduced-calorie diets challenging to adhere to in the long run. Furthermore, there's a decline in the levels of leptin, the satiety hormone. Reduced leptin can lead to increased appetite and diminished feelings of fullness after meals, again nudging one towards consuming more.

Additionally, the body becomes more efficient in its operations, meaning it learns to do the same tasks using fewer calories. For instance, the energy cost of walking a mile might decrease, so even with continued exercise, the caloric expenditure drops. Lastly, with reduced energy intake, there might be a decline in energy or motivation to engage in physical activity. This unintentional reduction in movement further decreases daily calorie burn. In essence, while reducing calorie intake seems like a straightforward method for weight loss, the body's multifaceted response system can counteract these efforts, making sustained weight loss a more nuanced endeavour than simple arithmetic.

The New Insight - The Carbohydrate-Insulin Model

A new theory called the Carbohydrate-Insulin Model flips the old idea on its head. Instead of saying that overeating causes weight gain, it suggests that how our body stores fat causes us to eat more. When we eat foods that are quickly turned into sugar in our bloodstream (like white bread or sugary drinks), our body releases insulin. This hormone pushes energy into fat storage, leaving less for our body to use. This makes us hungry and lowers our energy levels. Over time, this can lead to gradual weight gain.

Proof from Experiments

There have been numerous studies that support this new way of thinking. For example:

1. When rats were given foods that quickly turned to sugar, they stored more fat even if they ate the same amount of calories.

2. People seem to burn more calories when they eat fewer carbohydrates.

3. Certain medicines that affect insulin levels also impact weight.

Our blood glucose levels rise after consuming foods, particularly those abundant in rapidly digestible carbohydrates (such as sugary beverages and many processed foods). These carbohydrates are metabolised into glucose, the body's primary energy source. This surge in blood glucose prompts the pancreas to release insulin, a hormone essential for directing cells to absorb glucose. While it facilitates glucose absorption for energy, insulin simultaneously acts to store any excess glucose as fat. Beyond this, insulin impedes the breakdown of fat in our adipose tissues, effectively locking away our body's energy reserves.

The Carbohydrate-Insulin Model (CIM) suggests that a consistent intake of high-glycemic foods leads to persistently elevated insulin levels, making our bodies adept at fat storage. As more energy is siphoned into fat cells, fewer calories remain accessible for other bodily functions. This metabolic shift can paradoxically induce feelings of hunger, even if one's caloric intake is abundant. This heightened hunger can trigger further consumption of quickly digestible carbs, creating a vicious cycle of increased insulin production, enhanced fat storage, and recurrent hunger pangs.

In addition to these biological processes, a high-carbohydrate diet can cause shifts in energy partitioning, directing energy towards fat storage and away from other metabolic needs. This phenomenon, wherein the body feels energy-deprived despite adequate or even excessive caloric intake, highlights the potential pitfalls of focusing solely on calorie count without considering the source of those calories.

By reducing the intake of high-glycemic carbohydrates, we can moderate insulin spikes, stabilise blood sugar levels, and prevent excessive fat storage. This approach holds promise for weight management and offers a broader perspective on how our dietary choices impact overall metabolic health.

Insulin: The Sneaky Weight Gainer in the Hormonal Symphony of Fat

Have you ever wondered why men and women tend to accumulate fat differently? It turns out that male sex hormones play a significant role in inhibiting the type of fat accumulation commonly seen in women. When men are castrated, they often develop a fat distribution pattern that resembles that of women. This pattern is also observed in obese boys whose bodies haven't yet produced sufficient testicular hormones to prevent the accumulation of female-type adipose tissues. Surprisingly, female sex hormones also play a significant role in determining fat distribution. These hormones influence not just the distribution but also the quantity of fat, which explains the tendency for women to gain weight after menopause. Women who have their ovaries removed gain fat, much like postmenopausal women.

But there's more to the story. Insulin, the hormone responsible for regulating glucose levels in the blood, also has a role in fat deposition. It enhances the storage of glucose in adipose tissues and increases their affinity for accumulating fat. Obesity was once believed to result from genetic disorders affecting the hormonal regulation of fat metabolism. The process of converting food into fat is controlled by various enzymes, which are, in turn, regulated by hormones. Sex hormones determine where fat is stored, leading to the different fat distribution between men and women. Other hormones like thyroid hormone, adrenaline, and growth hormone play roles in releasing fatty acids from fat deposits, while insulin promotes fat storage. Obesity, it appears, is rooted in metabolic dysfunction.

The pivotal role of insulin as the "fattening hormone" became apparent after the discovery of type 1 diabetes. Women with type 1 diabetes, lacking insulin, remained thin despite increased appetite, while obese patients exhibited consistently high insulin levels. This revelation highlighted insulin's potential involvement in weight gain.

Deciphering Fat Storage: The Role of Insulin and Lipoprotein Lipase (LPL)

In the 1970s, researchers delved deep into the hormonal influences on body fat distribution, spotlighting the pivotal enzyme, Lipoprotein lipase (LPL). Dubbed the "fat's gatekeeper," LPL acts on circulating triglyceride-rich lipoproteins, converting them into fatty acids. These are either channelled for energy use by cells or designated for fat storage. Intriguingly, insulin, a hormone originating from the pancreas, dictates LPL's activity, but its influence varies across tissues. For instance, in adipose tissue, insulin amplifies LPL activity, but it diminishes it in muscular tissues. This nuanced regulation by insulin and other hormones deciphers the patterns of fat distribution, its gender-based differences, and its dynamic shifts with ageing and during phases like menopause.

Beyond its famed role in blood sugar management, insulin commands the conversion of carbohydrates into fats. This pancreatic hormone can surge fat production in the liver, raising both blood triglyceride and cholesterol levels. In our digestive tract, consumed carbohydrates break down primarily into glucose and fructose. On absorption, a rise in blood glucose propels the pancreas to discharge insulin. This hormone then steers tissues, especially the heart, muscles, and fat deposits, to take in these sugars, balancing blood sugar in the process. While a fraction of this sugar reserves as glycogen, an overload is redirected for fat formation, with insulin as the director. In the liver, it triggers lipogenesis, transforming sugars into acetyl coenzyme A, which subsequently becomes triglycerides and cholesterol.

These newly minted fats are then encased in very low-density lipoproteins (VLDL) by the liver and dispatched into our bloodstream. Organs like the heart, muscles, and fatty tissues mainly absorb these fats. To illustrate, the heart relies on triglycerides for up to 70% of its energy, while muscles tap into them during prolonged workouts. It's noteworthy that superfluous carbohydrate-derived calories often find their way to the midriff, manifesting as belly fat. A linchpin in lipid metabolism, LPL is vested with the role of hydrolysing triacylglycerol (TG) in TG-rich lipoproteins, aiding the delivery of fatty acids to various tissues. It is this collaborative working of insulin and LPL, with a special nod to the latter, that demystifies the body's adeptness at processing and stockpiling energy from ingested carbohydrates.

Battle of the Sexes: Decoding Fat Distribution

Women have more LPL activity in their adipose tissue than men, contributing to the higher prevalence of obesity in women. Men exhibit greater LPL activity in abdominal tissue, resulting in the classic "beer belly." Women, on the other hand, accumulate fat in the hips and buttocks, although after menopause, their abdominal LPL activity catches up with that of men. These variations in fat deposits are regulated by shifting levels of sex hormones. For instance, testosterone suppresses LPL activity in abdominal fat but has little impact on LPL in the lower body. The female hormones progesterone and oestrogen affect LPL differently, with progesterone increasing activity in the hips and buttocks and oestrogen reducing it. The decrease in oestrogen secretion during menopause, leading to increased LPL activity, may explain why women often gain weight during this life stage. This hormonal shift also accounts for changes in fat deposition during and after pregnancy.

Menopause, Carbs, and Confidence: Your Winning Combo

For women approaching menopause, managing insulin secretion by adopting a low-carbohydrate diet may be the key to maintaining a healthy weight. Keeping insulin levels low could be the solution, eliminating the need for restrictive or hunger-inducing diets. Additionally, a higher protein intake may promote better muscle maintenance, which becomes crucial during menopause.

Understanding the interplay between hormones, fat distribution, and diet can help women navigate the challenges of weight management during and after menopause. By keeping insulin levels in check and making strategic dietary choices, women can achieve their health goals without resorting to unsustainable or calorie-restrictive diets.

Essentially, the amount of time spent with insulin levels below a critical threshold—whether through time-restricted eating, intermittent fasting, or a low-carb, high-fat diet—determines whether the body mobilises or stores fat. For women approaching menopause, the key to success may lie in keeping insulin low, allowing for efficient fat-burning, and potentially entering a state of ketosis.

The conventional wisdom of adopting a low-calorie, low-fat diet for health beyond menopause is unsustainable and may lead to long-term issues like muscle loss and rebound weight gain.

Consider this: consuming a high-carb breakfast before a morning workout may seem like a good way to burn fat, but it's biologically impossible. Elevated insulin levels triggered by the carb-heavy meal inhibit fat burning. Moreover, grains contain lectins that bind to insulin receptors, further spiking blood sugar levels and signalling the body to store five times more fat. The result? It is an uphill battle against fat accumulation, even with exercise.

Reducing insulin secretion through a low-carb, not low-fat, diet can help women approaching menopause shed excess weight without the pitfalls of restrictive diets. Plus, it can mitigate the risk of sarcopenia—a condition where muscle mass is lost.

And there's a bonus: keeping blood glucose levels stable can also promote healthy, youthful-looking skin by preventing glycation, which leads to the formation of wrinkles and advanced glycation end products (AGEs). It's like creating your own metabolic heaven where weight management and skin health harmoniously coexist.

In conclusion, the key to metabolic heaven for women approaching menopause lies in insulin suppression through a low-carb, high-protein, and moderate-to-high-fat diet. This approach offers a sustainable solution to maintaining muscle mass and achieving lasting weight management without the burden of extreme diets. You will read more about this in the upcoming chapters.

Chapter Seven

The Hormonal Tango: Menopause and Insulin Resistance

Insulin Resistance (IR) is characterized by a body's weakened response to both its own insulin and insulin introduced from external sources. This impaired reaction results in decreased sensitivity of body tissues to insulin, subsequently leading to elevated blood glucose levels and an increased production of atherogenic lipids in the liver.

Menopause, which signifies the conclusion of a woman's reproductive phase, introduces a myriad of physiological changes, one of which is an increased predisposition to insulin resistance. This period witnesses a shift in fat distribution in women, transitioning from a gynoid (located around the hips and thighs) to an android (central abdominal) pattern. Consequently, while the overall percentage of body fat might remain constant, there's a significant augmentation in the intra-abdominal fat.

Role of Adiponectin

Adiponectin, a hormone secreted by fat cells, is known for its beneficial role in enhancing insulin sensitivity. It encourages cells to respond more effectively to insulin's signals, thereby facilitating efficient glucose uptake and utilisation. Elevated levels of adiponectin typically correlate with better metabolic health. However, post-menopausal women often experience a decline in adiponectin levels, potentially due to changes in fat distribution and increased central adiposity. This decline can exacerbate insulin resistance, a condition where cells no longer respond adequately to insulin's directives.

Insulin Dynamics After Menopause

The post-menopausal phase often witnesses an altered insulin dynamic. The accumulation of visceral fat, a characteristic change post-menopause, secretes inflammatory molecules that can impair insulin signalling. With suboptimal adiponectin levels to counterbalance this effect, the risk of insulin resistance escalates. Insulin resistance means the body needs more insulin to achieve the same glucose-lowering effect, leading to hyperinsulinemia. Chronic hyperinsulinemia can further suppress adiponectin production, creating a vicious cycle.

Implications of Insulin Resistance

When unchecked, insulin resistance paves the way for a spectrum of metabolic disorders, including type 2 diabetes, cardiovascular diseases, and fatty liver. Post-menopausal women, owing to hormonal and metabolic shifts, are particularly susceptible. Reduced adiponectin levels and increased central fat accumulation work in tandem, making post-menopausal women more vulnerable to these conditions.

In conclusion, understanding the interplay between adiponectin and insulin, especially in menopause, is pivotal. It underscores the importance of targeted interventions, like dietary adjustments and exercise, that can potentially enhance adiponectin levels and improve insulin sensitivity, helping post-menopausal women maintain metabolic well-being amidst hormonal shifts.

The Perils of Insulin Resistance

Insulin resistance is a health condition with far-reaching consequences. It can lead to:

1. Type 2 Diabetes: Insulin resistance is a primary factor in the development of type 2 diabetes, resulting in elevated blood sugar levels.

2. Cardiovascular Issues: Those with insulin resistance face an increased risk of heart disease, high blood pressure, and abnormal cholesterol levels, fostering atherosclerosis.

3. Obesity: Difficulty in regulating and storing fat can lead to weight gain and obesity, particularly around the abdomen.

4. Metabolic Syndrome: Insulin resistance is a cornerstone of metabolic syndrome, comprising conditions like high blood pressure, high blood sugar, abnormal cholesterol, and abdominal obesity, elevating the risk of heart disease and type 2 diabetes.

5. Liver Problems: Fat accumulation in the liver due to insulin resistance can result in non-alcoholic fatty liver disease (NAFLD) and, in severe cases, liver inflammation and scarring (cirrhosis).

6. Kidney Disease: Insulin resistance can damage kidney blood vessels, increasing the risk of kidney problems and diseases.

7. Cognitive Decline: Some studies suggest a link between insulin resistance and cognitive decline, raising the risk of conditions like Alzheimer's.

8. Inflammation: Chronic inflammation associated with insulin resistance contributes to health issues such as arthritis and certain cancers.

Understanding these interconnected health risks is crucial. Addressing insulin resistance through lifestyle changes, like a healthy diet and regular physical activity, can mitigate these risks and improve overall health.

Unlocking the Connection: Insulin Resistance and the Obesity Puzzle

I have the privilege of working with a group of individuals who have endured a profound societal bias: those struggling with obesity. By the time they reach out to me, they've often faced immense hardship, including feelings of shame, guilt, and the sting of discrimination.

Unfortunately, many people, including some in the healthcare field, tend to place the blame squarely on these individuals. The prevailing belief is that they should simply exert more self-control, and their weight issues would magically vanish. This perception couldn't be further from the truth.

Let me make one thing abundantly clear: obesity is not a matter of lacking character or willpower. It's a complex disease, intricately tied to hormones, with insulin playing a leading role.

Most obese individuals are grappling with insulin resistance, a condition akin to a precursor of type 2 diabetes. Insulin, often called the gatekeeper of blood sugar, has a crucial job: ushering glucose into cells for energy use. However, when someone is insulin-resistant, this process falters.

Imagine insulin as the key to a cell's front door, unlocking it to allow glucose in. In the case of insulin resistance, this key doesn't fit quite right, making it difficult for glucose to enter the cell. But glucose can't linger in the bloodstream indefinitely; otherwise, we'd all experience diabetic crises after every meal.

To compensate for this resistance, the body revs up its insulin production. Insulin levels soar as it attempts to overcome this barrier, often keeping blood sugar within the normal range for years. Yet, this heroic effort can only last so long, and even elevated insulin levels can't prevent blood sugar from eventually rising. That's when diabetes emerges.

It might not come as a surprise that many of my patients deal with insulin resistance or diabetes. But wait, that's not all. Even before pre-diabetes is diagnosed, many individuals have elevated insulin levels due to insulin resistance for many years, even decades. Furthermore, it's been found that 16-25% of people with normal weight also experience insulin resistance. So, when you add it up, a significant portion of the population is dealing with this issue.

Now, let's talk about the trouble with insulin resistance. When insulin levels rise, the risk of developing type 2 diabetes increases significantly. But that's not all. Insulin also profoundly impacts our appetite and how our bodies store fat. It's essentially our body's fat-storage hormone. This connection makes it clear why insulin resistance is closely tied to conditions like obesity and metabolic disorders such as diabetes.

The Carb-Insulin Connection: Hunger, Fat Storage, and Control

But what if we could address the root of the problem and reduce the excess glucose that insulin has to manage? Let's break it down. Everything we eat falls into one of three categories: carbohydrates, proteins, or fats. Each of these has a distinct effect on our glucose and, consequently, insulin levels.

Carbohydrates cause our insulin and glucose levels to spike rapidly. Proteins have a more moderate impact. Now, look at what happens when we consume fat – virtually nothing, a flat line. This observation is crucial.

Let's apply this to a real-life scenario. Think back to the last time you had Chinese food. We all know the unwritten rules: you tend to overeat because your body's satiety signals take a while to kick in. Then, about an hour later, you're ravenous again. Why? Because the rice in that meal caused your glucose and insulin levels to skyrocket, triggering hunger, fat storage, and cravings.

If you're already dealing with insulin resistance and have higher insulin levels, you're likely to experience constant hunger. In summary, when you consume carbs, your glucose and insulin levels surge, increasing hunger and fat storage. It's a cycle we need to address.

Rethinking Carbs: A New Approach to Eating for Health

Whether you are approaching menopause with or without insulin resistance or Type 2 diabetes, what you eat is crucial. But here's the thing: the traditional advice might do more harm than good. Let's focus on type 2 diabetes for a moment. The standard recommendation is to consume 40 to 65 grams of carbohydrates per meal and more at snack times. Sounds like a lot, right? It is, especially when you consider what carbs do to our blood sugar and insulin levels.

Eating carbs essentially means consuming the very thing that's causing the problem in the first place. It might sound crazy, but at its core, diabetes is a condition of carbohydrate overload. The sugar in our blood can't enter our cells correctly, causing immediate issues and, over time, even more severe consequences. Insulin resistance, a hallmark of diabetes, is a condition where our bodies become intolerant to carbohydrates. So why do we continue to recommend them?

The American Diabetes Association guidelines admit there's inconclusive evidence to recommend a specific carbohydrate limit. Yet, they also acknowledge that carb intake is the single most significant factor affecting blood sugar levels and the need for medication. To make things more complicated, if you're on certain diabetic medications, you might be told to eat carbs to avoid your blood sugar dropping too low. It's a vicious cycle: eat carbs, take meds, eat more carbs to counteract the side effects, and so on.

What's even more concerning is that these guidelines don't emphasise the possibility of reversing type 2 diabetes. But the truth is, it can be reversed, especially when caught early. We need to change this approach, spreading the message that there's hope and practical advice to achieve it.

So, let's rethink carbs. First, we must understand that we don't actually need them. Our bodies can function just fine without a single gram of carbohydrates. We have essential amino acids (proteins) and essential fatty acids, but there's no such thing as an essential carbohydrate. We can make all the glucose we need through a process called gluconeogenesis. Despite this, we continue to recommend that patients get over half of their daily energy from carbs, which doesn't align with our nutritional needs.

It's time to flip the script. Carbs become the minority of our intake, not the majority. How does it work? When we cut down on carbs, our blood sugar levels decrease; if you are diabetic, you will require less insulin. As a result, your insulin levels drop rapidly. It's a whole new approach to managing type 2 diabetes and making a world of difference.

Low-Carb Living: The Delicious Path to Health

Let's break it down in simple terms. How does eating low-carb work? Well, first, let's clear up some misconceptions. Low-carb doesn't mean zero-carb, and it's not all about eating heaps of protein. These are common myths we need to dispel.

So, if we're cutting carbs, what takes their place? Remember, we've got three main types of nutrients: carbs, protein, and fat. If one goes down, another must go up. In this case, my patients eat plenty of fat. Yes, you heard it right, fat! Why? Because fat is not only delicious, but it's also incredibly satisfying. Plus, it's the only macronutrient that keeps our blood sugar and insulin levels in check, and that's crucial.

Now, let me share my simple rules for eating this way. These rules are even more vital if you struggle with insulin levels.

Rule 1: If it says "light," "low-fat," or "fat-free" on the label, leave it in the grocery store. They've removed the fat and added carbs and chemicals.

Rule 2: Eat real food—the golden rule of low-carb nutrition. Real food doesn't come in a box; you should recognise it as natural.

Rule 3: Enjoy what you eat. Don't force yourself to eat something you don't like. Eat when you're hungry, not just because the clock says so.

Rule 4: Avoid GPS – No Grains, no Potatoes, and no Sugar. Sugar, in particular, is a big no-no.

Rule 5: Now, about grains. Many foods claiming to be whole grains are heavily processed, and their fibre benefits are compromised. For those who are insulin-sensitive, eating real whole grains may be okay, but for the vast majority with insulin issues, it's best to avoid them.

What if you're one of the lucky ones without insulin problems? Can you still eat this way? Absolutely! Even if you don't need it for your health, cutting carbs can be a great choice. I made the switch myself, and I'm not insulin-resistant. So, rest assured, low-carb can benefit everyone, whether it's a necessity or just a smart dietary choice.

Chapter Eight

The Low-Carb Therapeutic Approach to Health

Challenging Carbohydrate Conventions: The Arctic Pioneers

The modern high-carb diets began to take shape when traditional hunting cultures were slowly fading away in the face of expanding European influences. Between 1850 and 1930, the consumption of carbohydrates became commonplace, spreading from the U.S. Plains States through central Canada. Indigenous people in these regions had previously relied primarily on fat and protein and only sporadically used carbohydrates. Yet, the last group to uphold their traditional diet—the Inuit people of the Canadian and Alaskan Arctic—provided a unique glimpse into how a virtually carb-free diet could sustain them.

This dichotomy between scientific consensus and real-world observations presents an intriguing puzzle. In this chapter, we'll dive into the accounts of early explorer-scientists who interacted with the Inuit people, explore the controversies they stirred among nutritionists, and uncover forgotten lessons from the Inuit culture. These lessons may help us understand how well-being and physical performance can thrive without significant dietary carbohydrates.

The Dawn of Carbohydrate Dominance

Before the advent of agriculture, our ancestors consumed carbohydrates opportunistically. As some groups transitioned to hunting and fishing for sustenance, they ventured into temperate and arctic regions where access to grains, nuts, and fruits was limited. Fat and protein became their primary dietary energy sources in these harsh environments.

The rise of agriculture, which enabled the cultivation and storage of grains, allowed societies to establish permanent settlements and fostered the growth of written language. Wheat and rice-based cultures, originating in the Middle East and Asia, gradually spread over millennia to dominate Europe, Africa, and the Americas. Agricultural societies enjoyed the benefits of a sedentary lifestyle, higher population density, and permanent communities, which gave them an edge over hunting-based cultures.

Scientific nutrition studies in the early 20th century overwhelmingly supported carbohydrate's role as a necessary nutrient for human health and performance. A classic study in 1939 by Danish scientists

Christensen and Hansen emphasised the superiority of high-carb diets in enhancing endurance for high-intensity exercise. Another notable study during World War II investigated the practicality of pemmican, a meat and fat mixture, as an emergency ration. Soldiers subjected to a sudden switch from carbohydrate-containing rations to pemmican quickly became unable to perform physically demanding tasks.

The 1960s saw the development of percutaneous needle biopsy, allowing researchers to delve into muscle fuel stores and metabolism. This led to the concept that muscle glycogen was the critical fuel for high-intensity exercise, giving rise to carbohydrate-loading strategies. The consensus was that fat had limited use as an exercise fuel, and a low-carb diet was believed to impair physical performance.

The Hunter's Perspective: Insights from Ketogenic Diets

While high-carb diets may excel in short-term high-intensity tests, numerous hints in the literature suggest that the drawbacks of ketogenic diets might be exaggerated. Historical evidence reveals that entire populations thrived for millennia as hunters, challenging the notion that carbohydrates are essential for survival.

One remarkable example is the Schwatka expedition of 1878–80. This expedition covered over 3000 miles on foot across ice, snow, and tundra with limited supplies, relying solely on hunting and fishing for food. Lt. Frederick Schwatka, a U.S. Army surgeon, noted an initial weakness when transitioning from a carbohydrate-rich diet to one based on reindeer meat. However, within a few weeks, this weakness vanished, demonstrating the body's adaptability to a low-carb diet.

Vilhjalmur Stefansson, a Harvard-trained anthropologist, ventured into the Arctic in the early 1900s to study Inuit culture. He found himself living with Inuit groups for extended periods, adopting their hunter's diet. Stefansson's accounts sparked controversy, as he claimed that humans could thrive solely on meat and fat, challenging prevailing nutrition wisdom.

In 1929, Stefansson conducted a year-long experiment with a colleague, consuming only meat and fat under scientific observation. Contrary to expectations, they remained healthy throughout the experiment, dispelling fears of scurvy and other deficiencies. This study revealed that a high-fat, moderate-protein diet could sustain individuals.

It's essential to note that the Inuit diet primarily consisted of fat, with a moderate protein intake. Stefansson observed that the Inuit deliberately reserved lean meat for their dogs, highlighting their preference for the higher-fat portions.

Intriguingly, Stefansson's defence of his findings likely played a role in developing carbohydrate-loading strategies. His advocacy of pemmican (mixture of tallow, dried meat, and sometimes dried berries) as an emergency ration during World War II led to the Kark study and subsequent dietary trials.

The clash between conventional nutritional wisdom and the experiences of cultures living on low-carb diets raises important questions. Can humans adapt to thrive without significant dietary carbohydrates, as the Inuit did? Our history, exploration, and scientific discovery journey offers insights into this enduring mystery. As we delve deeper into the intriguing world of nutrition and endurance, we'll continue to explore the remarkable resilience of the human body when faced with dietary challenges.

The Ketogenic Diet: From Medical Origins to Modern Weight Loss Craze

The ketogenic diet, often referred to as "keto," is a dietary approach that has a fascinating history. Initially, it emerged as a medical treatment in the 19th century, primarily for managing diabetes. Fast forward to the 1920s, and it gained recognition as an effective therapy for epilepsy, particularly in children when traditional medications fell short. Over the years, the ketogenic diet hasn't been limited to just these medical uses; it has also been explored as a therapeutic approach for conditions like cancer, diabetes, polycystic ovary syndrome (PCOS), and Alzheimer's disease.

However, what's caught the attention of many in recent times is the keto diet's potential for weight loss. This surge in popularity can be partly attributed to the low-carb diet trend that began in the 1970s with the Atkins diet. The Atkins diet, known for its very low-carbohydrate, high-fat approach, achieved commercial success and significantly contributed to popularising low-carb diets. Today, other low-carb diets such as Paleo, South Beach, and Dukan have gained popularity. These diets also emphasise protein but maintain a moderate fat intake. The ketogenic diet, on the other hand, stands out due to its distinctive high-fat content, typically making up 70% to 80% of total daily calories, with protein intake kept at a moderate level.

Ketosis Explained: The Science Behind the Ketogenic Diet's Weight Loss Mechanism

The ketogenic diet's weight loss principle revolves around altering the body's primary source of energy. Normally, our cells rely on glucose, obtained from carbohydrates in our diet, as their main fuel. However, when carbohydrates are severely restricted, an alternative energy source kicks in: ketones. This switch is what gives the diet its name, "ketogenic."

The brain has a constant demand for glucose, about 120 grams daily, as it cannot store this energy source. When there's a lack of glucose due to fasting or minimal carbohydrate intake, the body initially taps into stored glucose in the liver and even breaks down muscle tissue to release glucose. If this continues for 3-4 days and stored glucose is fully depleted, blood levels of insulin, a hormone that regulates glucose, drop. This prompts the body to use fat as its main energy source primarily. The liver starts producing ketone bodies from fat, which can be used in the absence of glucose.

When ketone bodies accumulate in the blood, this state is known as ketosis. It's important to clarify that ketosis is a mild and natural condition, often experienced by healthy individuals during periods of fasting, such as overnight sleep or strenuous exercise. Proponents of the ketogenic diet argue that if the diet is carefully followed, blood ketone levels should not reach a harmful level, as the brain can use ketones as fuel. Healthy individuals typically produce enough insulin to prevent excessive ketone production.

The onset of ketosis and the level of ketone bodies in the blood can vary from person to person. It depends on factors like body fat percentage and resting metabolic rate.

Ketosis vs. Ketoacidosis: Understanding the Key Differences

The Ketone Zone: Nutritional Ketosis versus DKA

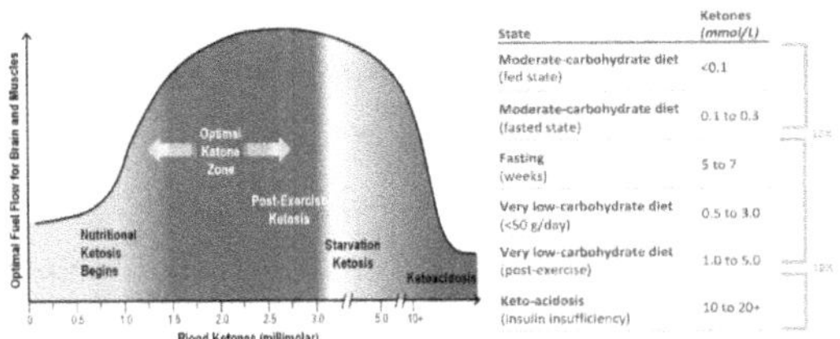

Source Dr. Stephen Phinney

It's essential to distinguish between ketosis and ketoacidosis. While ketosis is a natural and harmless state, ketoacidosis is a potentially dangerous condition. Ketoacidosis occurs when there is an excessive accumulation of ketone bodies in the blood, resulting in a dangerously high acid level. This condition is more common in individuals with type 1 diabetes because they do not produce insulin, a hormone that helps regulate ketone levels. In rare cases, ketoacidosis has been reported in non-diabetic individuals following an extended period of very low-carbohydrate dieting.

Ketogenic Diet Essentials: Low-Carb Foods & Guidelines

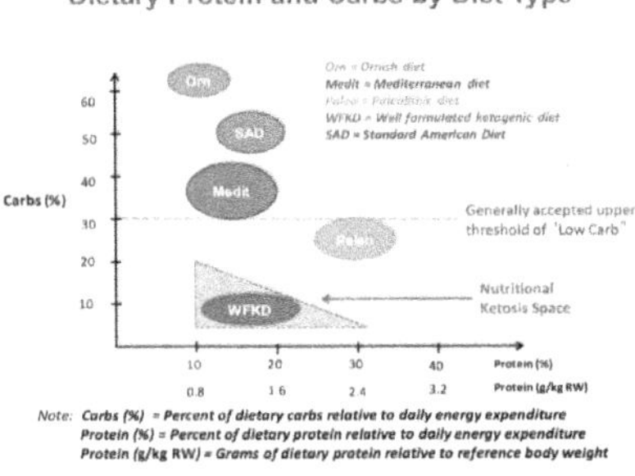

Source Dr. Stephen Phinney

The ketogenic diet typically involves reducing daily carbohydrate intake to less than 50 grams, equivalent to the amount found in a medium plain bagel. It can sometimes be as low as 20 grams per day. On the ketogenic diet, I often recommend an average of 70% to 80% of daily calories from fat, 5% to 10% from carbohydrates, and 10% to 15% from protein. Protein intake is kept moderate at about 1.5g/kg to prevent it from interfering with ketosis since excess protein can be converted into glucose, potentially disrupting the state of ketosis. While the ketogenic diet is known for its high fat content, it's important to maintain protein intake to preserve lean body mass, including muscle. (see figure diagram above)

Variations of the ketogenic diet exist, but they all share the characteristic of eliminating carb-rich foods. Some obvious carb sources include bread, pasta, rice, and sugary snacks. However, certain foods you might not immediately associate with carbohydrates, like beans, legumes, and most fruits, are also restricted. On the flip side, the diet typically allows foods high in saturated fat, including fatty cuts of meat, processed meats, lard, and butter. It also includes sources of unsaturated fats like nuts, seeds, avocados, plant oils, and fatty fish.

Here is a list of all the low-carb foods that are appropriate to eat when you're following a ketogenic diet.

1. Fish and seafood

2. Low-carb veggies

3. Cheese

4. Avocados

5. Poultry

6. Eggs

7. Nuts, seeds and healthful oils

8. Plain Greek yoghurt and cottage cheese

9. Berries

10. Unsweetened coffee and tea

11. Dark chocolate and cocoa powder

Decoding the Science: Ketogenic Diet Research Insights

Research into the ketogenic diet has shown promising metabolic changes in the short term. Alongside weight loss, improvements have been observed in health markers associated with excess weight, such as insulin resistance, high blood pressure, and elevated cholesterol and triglyceride levels. There's also growing interest in using low-carbohydrate diets, including the ketogenic diet, for managing type 2 diabetes. Several theories exist about why the ketogenic diet might promote weight loss, although they haven't been consistently confirmed in research:

1. Satiety: The high-fat content of the diet may reduce food cravings.

2. Hormone Regulation: Eating limited carbs may lead to a decrease in appetite-stimulating hormones like insulin and ghrelin.

3. Ketone Bodies: These may directly reduce hunger while serving as the body's primary fuel source.

4. Increased Calorie Expenditure: Converting fat and protein into glucose may boost calorie burning.

5. Fat Loss: Lower insulin levels may encourage fat loss rather than muscle loss.

Now, let's delve into the findings of research specific to the ketogenic diet. The studies included in this list focused on diets that consisted of about 70% to 80% fat, 10% to 20% protein, and 5% to 10% carbohydrates. It's important to note that some diets referred to as "low carbohydrate" may not adhere to these specific ratios, potentially allowing higher protein or carbohydrate intake. For this discussion, we are concentrating on studies related to obesity or overweight individuals.

1. *Meta-analysis of Weight Loss*: A meta-analysis of 13 randomised controlled trials tracked overweight and obese participants for 1-2 years. The study compared low-fat diets with very low-carbohydrate ketogenic diets. The results showed that the ketogenic diet led to a small but significantly greater reduction in weight, triglycerides, and blood pressure compared to the low-fat diet at one year. However, the authors noted that the difference in weight loss between the two diets was about 2 pounds and that compliance with the ketogenic diet declined over time. This decline in compliance may have contributed to the more significant difference at one year but not at two years.

2. *Appetite Regulation*: A systematic review of 26 short-term intervention trials (lasting 4-12 weeks) assessed the appetites of overweight and obese individuals. These individuals followed either a very low-calorie diet (~800 calories daily) or a ketogenic diet (no calorie restriction but ≤50 grams of carbohydrates daily). None of the studies directly compared the two diets; instead, they measured participants' appetites before and after the diet periods. Despite significant weight loss on both diets, participants reported reduced hunger and a decreased desire to eat on the ketogenic diet compared to baseline measurements. Surprisingly, there was no increase in hunger, even with the extreme dietary restrictions. Researchers attributed this to changes in

appetite hormones like ghrelin and leptin, as well as the presence of ketone bodies and increased fat and protein intake.

3. *Obese Adults on a Ketogenic Diet*: A study involving 39 obese adults placed on a ketogenic, very low-calorie diet for 8 weeks. The results showed an average loss of 13% of their initial weight, accompanied by significant reductions in fat mass, insulin levels, blood pressure, and waist and hip measurements. Notably, their levels of ghrelin, the hunger hormone, did not increase during ketosis, contributing to a reduced appetite. However, during the 2-week period when participants returned to a normal diet, their ghrelin levels and urges to eat significantly increased.

4. *Ketogenic Diet vs. Mediterranean Diet*: A study involving 89 obese adults implemented a two-phase diet plan. The participants followed a very low-carbohydrate ketogenic diet for 6 months, followed by a 6-month reintroduction phase on a normal-calorie Mediterranean diet. This study demonstrated a significant mean weight loss of 10% with no weight regain after one year. The ketogenic diet in this study provided approximately 980 calories per day, with 12% from carbohydrates, 36% from protein, and 52% from fat. In contrast, the Mediterranean diet offered about 1800 calories daily, with 58% from carbohydrates, 15% from protein, and 27% from fat. Remarkably, 88% of the participants adhered to the entire regimen. It's worth noting that the ketogenic diet used in this study contained lower fat and slightly higher carbohydrate and protein levels compared to the standard ketogenic diet, which typically provides 70% or more of daily calories from fat and less than 20% from protein.

Embarking on the Keto Adventure: Your Weight Loss Journey Begins Here

Here's how a ketogenic diet works when you want to shed some pounds: Your appetite naturally decreases, allowing you to consume fewer calories than you burn—this calorie deficit results in weight loss. Interestingly, your body fat contributes to the energy you need alongside the calories from the food you eat. So, even though it may appear that you're consuming more protein and fat, a significant portion of your energy comes from your stored body fat.

As you progress in your weight loss journey, your metabolism may slow down slightly due to reduced body mass. You might find that your appetite returns and your rate of weight loss decreases. However, if you maintain a low-carb lifestyle and embrace dietary fats, you can continue to lose weight more sustainably. The key is not to fear fats but to incorporate them into your daily meals.

This approach allows you to transition from weight loss to maintenance without the risk of regaining lost pounds. It's a lifestyle change that can lead to improved health, sustained weight loss, and potentially, a longer and healthier life.

Saturated vs. Monounsaturated Fats: Deciphering Your Body's Preferred Fuel

We've often been cautioned about saturated fats, but let's set the record straight. Saturated fats are in the red corner, while the preferred fuel for your body, monounsaturated fats, sits in the yellow corner. When your body predominantly uses fat for energy, these monounsaturated fats take the lead. Why? We won't dive too deep into the science, but trust us, it's your body's way of saying, "I like this fuel."

Monounsaturated fats are found in high concentrations in olive oils, avocados, nuts such as almonds, hazelnuts, pecans, and seeds such as pumpkin and sesame seeds.

Saturated fats are found in animal-based foods like beef, pork, poultry, full-fat dairy products, eggs, and tropical oils like coconut and palm.

Omega-6 Overload: The Unsettling Truth About Common Cooking Oils

Polyunsaturated fatty acids (PUFAs) are a group of fats that contain more than one double bond in their chemical structure. These double bonds make PUFAs more chemically reactive compared to saturated fats, which have no double bonds. Due to these double bonds, PUFAs are more susceptible to oxidation, a chemical reaction where electrons are lost, often due to heat, light, or oxygen exposure. This oxidation process can produce harmful compounds known as reactive oxygen species (ROS), free radicals that can cause cellular damage. Oxidised PUFAs can contribute to inflammation and other health problems when consumed in large amounts. Therefore, while PUFAs have essential roles in our bodies, it's crucial to balance their intake and be cautious about exposing them to conditions that can lead to oxidation.

Within the family of PUFAs, there are two main categories: omega-3 and omega-6 fatty acids. Both are essential for human health, meaning the body cannot produce them, so they must be obtained through the diet.

Omega-6 fatty acids are a type of PUFA. Our diet's primary omega-6 fatty acid is linoleic acid, which can be converted to other omega-6 fatty acids in the body. Linoleic acid is found in high concentrations in many vegetable oils, such as safflower, sunflower, corn, soybean, and cottonseed.

While omega-6 fatty acids are essential for various physiological functions, including supporting skin health and producing pro-inflammatory molecules, the modern Western diet often contains an imbalanced ratio of omega-6 to omega-3 fatty acids. Historically, human diets had a ratio close to 1:1, but today's diets can have ratios as high as 15:1 or 20:1 in favour of omega-6.

Such a skewed ratio can promote an inflammatory environment in the body, which is believed to contribute to various chronic diseases. To support overall health, achieving a more balanced intake of omega-3 and omega-6 fatty acids is beneficial.

Now, when it comes to essential fats, the omega-6 family is in the spotlight. Yes, you need them, but only in small quantities – about a teaspoonful daily. The catch? Most of us get our fats from the "big blues": safflower, sunflower, corn, soybean, peanut, and cottonseed oils. These oils are high in omega-6 and can make you feel unwell. Picture bike racers refusing soybean oil after a week because it simply didn't agree with their stomachs. And, trust me, these racers usually have ironclad stomachs. Omega-3 fatty acids can be derived from fish and other seafood (especially cold-water fatty fish, such as salmon, mackerel, tuna, herring, and sardines), nuts and seeds (such as flaxseed, chia seeds, and walnuts).

Low-Carb Meal Guide

Now, let's talk about practicality. What does a typical low-carb meal look like? It's actually quite delicious. Here is a simple example of what I would eat in a day on a ketogenic diet.

Breakfast: Start your day with a cup of black coffee. You can even add a touch of butter if you prefer. Some folks like to use medium-chain fatty acids in their coffee, but butter works just as well. Pair it with a real sausage – no mystery meat here.

Lunch: Fill your plate with a generous helping of green vegetables and a hearty salad. Include about six ounces of water-packed tuna. To stay low in 'bad' fats, choose water-packed tuna instead of oil-packed. Make a rich dressing using olive oil or full-fat yoghurt to add the fats your body craves.

Snacks: Nuts and soft cheese make excellent snacks. Don't be afraid to indulge in these luscious options.

Dinner: Dinner can be a feast! Enjoy a flavorful meal that includes four ounces of homemade, full-fat ice cream – yes, you read that right, you can make it yourself. Pair it with tomato bisque made from fresh garden tomatoes and chicken broth, which is an essential part of this diet.

The Importance of Broth

Now, let's emphasise something crucial – broth. It's a cornerstone of this diet and comes from a traditional practice of many indigenous people. You'll want to consume two cups of broth or bouillon daily. This not only adds flavour but also provides you with essential sodium, which your body needs as it enters ketosis.

Here is my recipe for making a keto-friendly bone broth. I use an Instant Pot for making my Bone Broth because it is versatile and quick. With this kitchen marvel, you can prepare your bone broth using either the slow cooker or pressure cooking functions. Additionally, you have the option to sauté the bones before commencing your soup-making adventure, offering even more culinary flexibility.

Ingredients You'll Need:

- Olive Oil

- Beef Bones

- Kohlrabi

- Leek

- Carrots

- Onion

- Garlic

- Parsley

- Apple Cider Vinegar

Step One: Ingredient Preparation. Gather all your bones, thoroughly clean the vegetables, and cut them into larger pieces. Remember, the larger the pieces, the longer it will take for the veggies to cook and soften.

Step Two: Sautéing. Switch on the Instant Pot's Sauté function, add some olive oil, and toss in the bones for a good sauté from all angles.

Step Three: Add Veggies and Water. Introduce the vegetables, vinegar, herbs, salt, and pepper to the mix. Close the lid securely, ensuring the pressure valve is set to the closed position.

Step Four: Cooking. Select the soup function and set the timer for 2 hours on high pressure. After this, allow the Instant Pot to release pressure for optimal results naturally.

Step Five: Straining. Once the soup has cooled to a manageable temperature, strain it through a muslin cloth to obtain the clearest and purest broth possible.

The 7 Steps to Success

To ensure your low-carb journey is successful, remember these seven key steps:

1. Moderate Protein: Keep your protein intake moderate, not too high.

2. Energy from Fat: Once your weight stabilises, most of your energy should come from dietary fats.

3. The Right Fats: Choose your fats wisely, favouring the healthier options.

4. Salt Your Food: Lightly or moderately salt your food, and don't shy away from it. Your body needs it.

5. Broth Is Your Friend: Consume two cups of broth or bouillon each day to maintain proper mineral levels.

6. Monitor Ketones: Keep an eye on your blood ketone levels, and if they dip below the desired range, adjust your carb intake. You can monitor your ketone levels through various methods, but my favourite is using ketone metres. Another approach is using urinalysis strips, which test for ketones in urine. However, their accuracy may vary. For a non-invasive option, breath ketone metres measure acetone in your breath.

7. Enjoy Satiety and Variety: Find pleasure and satisfaction in your meals by exploring different flavours and textures. This will lead to better health and overall well-being.

In conclusion, a low-carb lifestyle isn't just about weight loss; it's about nurturing your body with the right fats while savouring delicious foods. It's a journey to lasting health, and you have the tools to make it work for you. So, embrace fats, enjoy your meals, and thrive on this low-carb adventure for years to come.

Chapter 9
Keto in Motion: Mastering Exercise on a Ketogenic Diet

Let's delve into a pivotal moment in my medical journey—a moment that led me to question the conventional wisdom surrounding carbohydrates and endurance. In the last few years, as we battled lockdowns and covid scares, I developed a fervour for running. I would eagerly hop into my running shoes whenever I could find a hill or slope and attempt to conquer it just to see if I could. What I learned during these runs would challenge my understanding of nutrition.

I discovered that when my diet was rich in carbohydrates and I consumed them during my runs, I could run for hours without any issues. However, if I refrained from consuming carbohydrates during a run lasting more than an hour, I would suddenly hit a figurative wall. This phenomenon, known as "hitting the wall," is common among endurance athletes. It occurs when they deplete their energy reserves during extended events due to insufficient carbohydrate intake, leading to a dramatic drop in performance.

As I engaged in discussions with sports nutritionists coaching professional athletes, we contemplated the impact of low-carb diets, like the Atkins diet (a high-fat, low-carb diet), on athletic performance. The prevailing belief was that such diets, devoid of carbohydrates, would hinder performance. However, some athletes who had adopted these diets reported that their athletic performance remained unaffected, even after months of low-carb living. This is when I started my research into ketogenic diets and performance. And I thought the best place to start was to see what the ultra-endurance athletes were doing. I have always said it is far better to compare yourself to the elite than to the average (which, in many cases, are sedentary individuals we are trying not to learn from).

Ketogenic Diets and Physical Performance: Debunking Myths with Science

In the 1970s, there was a growing interest in very low-calorie ketogenic diets, essentially low-carb and high-fat diets for weight loss. It was hypothesised that exercise tolerance might take longer to recover after removing carbohydrates from the diet. This idea was supported by Schwatka's observation that adaptation to a diet devoid of carbohydrates took several weeks.

To test this hypothesis, a study by Dr. Stephen Phinney under the guidance of Drs. Ethan Sims and Edward Horton at the University of Vermont was conducted. Participants followed a very low-calorie ketogenic diet for six weeks, with their protein and some inherent fat coming from lean meat, fish, and poultry. To ensure mineral balance, they were given supplemental sodium and potassium. Treadmill tests measured peak aerobic power and endurance time to exhaustion. Interestingly, despite a decrease in endurance after one week on the ketogenic diet, it significantly improved beyond baseline after six weeks, although the energy cost of exercise had decreased.

A second study by Dr. Phinney, under the mentorship of Dr. Bruce Bistrian at MIT, involved competitive bicycle racers. They followed a ketogenic diet patterned after Stefansson's, aiming to maintain ketosis without losing weight. These subjects experienced a temporary decline in energy during the first week of the diet, but their performance was reasonably restored, except for sprint capability, which remained limited.

The results of these studies demonstrated that, after an initial adjustment period, both untrained individuals and highly trained athletes could maintain or even improve their physical performance on a ketogenic diet. Notably, there was no loss of peak aerobic power despite the absence of dietary carbohydrates for extended periods.

Three factors help explain these findings:

1. Adaptation: Keto-adaptation takes longer than a week, likely extending to 3-4 weeks. It requires consistent adherence to carbohydrate restriction, and individuals who intermittently consume carbs while attempting a ketogenic diet often report reduced exercise tolerance.

2. Sodium and Potassium: Optimised mineral intake is crucial. The Inuit people, who traditionally consumed ketogenic diets, optimised their sodium and potassium intake, contributing to their ability to maintain physical performance. Providing adequate sodium and potassium through supplements helped maintain the circulatory reserve and functional tissue preservation in the studies.

3. Protein Dose: Adjusting protein intake within the range of 1.2 to 1.7 grams per kilogram of reference body weight daily, along with adequate minerals, preserving lean body mass and physical performance. Too little protein can lead to a loss of lean tissue, while excessive protein intake can suppress ketosis and lead to adverse effects.

In conclusion, observational and prospective studies indicate that a ketogenic diet can maintain submaximal endurance performance. However, successful implementation requires attention to keto-adaptation, mineral balance, and appropriate protein intake. While ketogenic diets may limit anaerobic performance, they should not hinder most forms of physical activity or labour, except under competitive athletics requiring high muscle glycogen levels.

Ketones & Athletic Excellence: Beyond Carbs and Combating Oxidative Stress

In one study, five athletes were put on a low-carb, high-fat diet for four weeks. The goal was to see how this diet affected their performance. The results were intriguing. While the average endurance time to exhaustion increased for most athletes, one person's performance improved significantly, another saw a moderate improvement, and two others experienced a decline. It became evident that our bodies react differently to dietary changes, showing that we are not all the same regarding nutrition.

There are two main takeaways from this study. First, it raised the question of whether four weeks of adaptation to a low-carb diet is sufficient for everyone. Some individuals may need more time to adapt to this dietary shift fully. Second, it's crucial to understand that transitioning from a high-carb diet to a high-fat one does not happen overnight. It requires consistent effort and dedication, not just a quick fix.

Now, you might wonder if adopting a low-carb diet could be dangerous. To answer this question, let's examine a study involving 40 people with metabolic syndrome (a precursor to diabetes). They were divided into two groups: one followed a low-fat diet, while the other followed a high-fat, low-carb diet rich in saturated fats. Surprisingly, the results showed that the group on the high-fat diet lost more weight, even though they consumed 36 grams of saturated fat per day compared to 12 grams in the low-fat group. This suggests that a low-carb, high-fat diet may not be as risky as it seems.

Several athletes have adopted this dietary approach as a lifestyle, not just a short-term strategy. They've achieved remarkable feats, breaking records and completing challenging races while fueling their bodies with fat rather than carbohydrates. For instance, Timothy Olson, a competitive ultrarunner, shattered records in a 100-mile race using a low-carb diet. A high school teacher, Zach Bitter ran 100 miles in under 12 hours on a similar diet. Even an army sergeant, Mike Morton, set an American record for running 172 miles in 24 hours while following a low-carb diet.

These examples illustrate that a low-carb, high-fat diet can be a game-changer for athletes. It challenges traditional beliefs about the need for high carbohydrate intake and demonstrates that our bodies are incredibly adaptable.

The Ketone Chronicles: Unveiling the Power of Ketones

Understanding the concept of oxidative stress (OS) and its relationship with exercise is crucial. Oxidative stress refers to an imbalance between the production of harmful free radicals, known as reactive oxygen species (ROS), and the body's ability to neutralise them using antioxidants. When ROS overwhelms our antioxidant defence systems, it becomes a significant factor in various chronic diseases like diabetes, heart disease, and possibly cancer.

A Battle Within— ROS vs. Antioxidants: Because of their rigorous training routines, Ultra-endurance athletes generate an immense quantity of reactive oxygen species. These athletes often struggle to maintain balance in the face of this oxidative onslaught. The result? Signs of overtraining and the body's inability to cope with the flood of free radicals.

Ketones to the Rescue: Recent research has unveiled a promising ally against oxidative stress: ketones. These compounds, produced during a ketogenic diet, offer protection against oxidative stress and enhance the body's antioxidant defence system. This discovery holds implications not only for athletes but also for individuals with various clinical diseases and disorders.

The Anti-Inflammatory Effect of Ketones: Ketones don't stop at just reducing oxidative stress; they also exhibit anti-inflammatory properties. Scientists have uncovered the underlying mechanisms through which ketones, such as those in a ketogenic diet, can suppress inflammation. A key player in this process is the NLRP3 inflammasome, a molecular complex involved in inflammatory responses.

Human Evidence of Ketone Power: Human trials have provided tangible evidence of ketones' anti-inflammatory effects. In a study involving patients with metabolic syndrome, those on a ketogenic diet for 12 weeks experienced a reduction in pro-inflammatory cytokines and adhesion molecules, surpassing the results of a low-fat diet group.

Taming Inflammation in Type 2 Diabetes: In individuals with type 2 diabetes who adopted a ketogenic diet, a year-long journey yielded remarkable results. These participants experienced a significant decrease in white blood cell count, a reliable indicator of inflammation. High-sensitive C-reactive protein, another inflammation marker, dropped by an impressive 39%.

The Swift Recovery Advantage: One of the most tangible benefits reported by athletes who embrace a ketogenic diet is their ability to recover swiftly and entirely after strenuous exercise. Ultra-endurance athletes who've made the switch often feel remarkably well the day after running long distances, despite the typical fatigue and muscle soreness following such endeavours. This accelerated recovery can be attributed to reduced oxidative stress and inflammation, as evidenced by elevated markers after ultra-endurance runs. Why are we interested in studying endurance athletes? Well, we know that what can work for them can also work for menopausal women looking to optimise their health and exercise performance.

The Bonk-Proof Brain: Ketogenic adaptation provides unique neurological protection, rendering the brain nearly "bonk-proof." Hitting the wall, a state of catastrophic fatigue during prolonged exercise, is primarily an energy crisis in the brain. Ketone-adapted athletes seem impervious to this crisis thanks to lower oxidative stress and inflammation. This newfound neural protection ensures consistent cognitive function and resilience during physically demanding activities.

Ketones: A Fuel for the Brain and Heart: Both the brain and the heart readily uptake ketones as an alternative fuel source. This metabolic flexibility is especially beneficial in times of glucose scarcity, offering protection from hypoglycemia. Moreover, the heart prefers ketones even at lower concentrations, highlighting their role as a valuable energy source for this vital organ.

Unlocking the Power of Ketones for Health and Performance

First, it's essential to understand how our bodies use different fuels for energy. Traditionally, we've been taught that carbohydrates are our primary source of energy, especially for our brains. However, recent research challenges this notion, introducing us to the concept of ketones.

Ketones are molecules produced by our bodies when we shift from primarily burning carbohydrates to burning fat for fuel. This metabolic state is known as ketosis. But don't confuse it with ketoacidosis, a dangerous condition that can occur in uncontrolled diabetes. Ketosis is a controlled and healthy state that can have numerous benefits.

So, how do we enter ketosis? One way is through a well-formulated low-carb, high-fat diet. This approach restricts carbohydrate intake while increasing fat consumption. When you eat this way, your body starts to break down fat into ketones, which can be used for energy. Another way is to use fasting which I will discuss later in Chapter 10.

Ketogenic Diets & Heart Health: Challenging Traditional Beliefs with Surprising Outcomes

Now, let's explore the impact of a ketogenic diet on health. In a study involving two groups of individuals—one following a low-carb, high-fat diet, and the other a low-fat diet—the results were eye-opening. The low-carb group experienced more significant weight loss than the low-fat group. But what about heart health?

One crucial marker for heart health is LDL cholesterol, often referred to as "bad cholesterol." Surprisingly, LDL cholesterol increased slightly in the low-carb group but decreased in the low-fat group.

However, these changes were small and not statistically significant. What's more important than LDL levels is the size of LDL particles. A three percent increase in particle size can significantly reduce the risk of heart disease. This increase was observed in the low-carb group, indicating a potential reduction in risk.

But that's not all. The low-carb group also saw substantial improvements in HDL cholesterol, known as "good cholesterol," and a remarkable 50% reduction in triglycerides. This reduction in the HDL to triglycerides ratio is a promising indicator of improved metabolic health.

Now, here's where it gets fascinating. Researchers measured the amount of saturated fat circulating in the bloodstream. You might think eating more saturated fat would increase these levels, but the opposite happened. Despite consuming three times as much saturated fat as the low-fat group, the low-carb group had lower levels of saturated fat in their blood. How can this be?

The key lies in our body's remarkable ability to adapt. When you follow a well-formulated low-carb diet and enhance your body's fat-burning capacity, saturated fat becomes a high-octane fuel that your body efficiently burns, reducing its accumulation in the bloodstream.

Ketones: The Brain's Ancient Fuel and the Athlete's Modern Edge

But what about ketones and their role in brain function? Traditionally, we believed that the brain relied heavily on glucose. However, when ketone levels rise in your body, the brain can derive over half of its energy from ketones, making it a powerful and efficient fuel source.

This shift in understanding ketones has opened new avenues for health and performance. Ketones aren't just an alternative fuel; they might be the primary fuel that our distant ancestors thrived on during times of scarcity.

In recent years, more and more athletes have explored the benefits of a ketogenic diet. These athletes have crossed finish lines, shattered records, and achieved remarkable feats while fueling their bodies primarily with ketones. So if you are exercising while on a ketogenic diet, you can take a leaf from these athletes so that you can be adequately fueled from ketones as long as you are keto-adapted, and that may take weeks to months depending on your metabolic health and adaptation mechanisms.

Unlocking Longevity: The Power of Beta-Hydroxybutyrate

Beta-Hydroxybutyrate (BHB) is one of the three ketone bodies produced by the liver, primarily from fatty acids, during periods of low food intake, carbohydrate-restrictive diets, or prolonged intense exercise. The liver breaks down fats to produce fatty acids when glucose availability is limited. These fatty acids are then converted into acetyl-CoA, which enters the liver's mitochondria. Within the mitochondria, some of the acetyl-CoA is used to produce BHB. Once formed, BHB can be released into the bloodstream and transported to various tissues, particularly the brain, to be used as a primary energy source in the absence of glucose.

In a groundbreaking study published in the prestigious journal Science, a group of researchers from San Francisco uncovered various health benefits of BHB. Here's the exciting part: BHB acts like a messenger that goes straight to the nucleus of our cells, where our genetic instructions reside. Specifically, it influences a group of genes known as histone deacetylases. These genes play a vital role in our body's defence against harmful substances called free radicals, often associated with oxidative stress. When BHB levels rise, it's like turning on a powerful shield against oxidative stress and free radicals. Imagine it as taking a super-potent antioxidant, but the magic happens from within your own body.

Now, let's flip the script and look at our recent ancestors who shifted towards agriculture and started consuming copious amounts of carbohydrates. Their BHB levels dropped significantly, which means their natural defences against oxidative stress got weakened. This might explain why we've developed a need for external antioxidants like those found in foods such as spinach.

But the story doesn't end there. Recent research has linked BHB to other health benefits, including stabilising mast cells, which play a role in allergies and asthma. Many individuals with upper airway issues have reported significant improvements when adopting a low-carb diet. We now have a biological mechanism that explains this phenomenon.

Perhaps the most intriguing revelation comes from studying tiny creatures known as C. elegans or nematodes. These creatures are used in longevity research to discover substances that can extend life without harmful side effects. When researchers introduced BHB into their environment, these nematodes lived an astonishing 26% longer. This exciting finding has triggered a rush of interest from longevity researchers in low-carb diets.

Increasing the body's Beta-Hydroxybutyrate (BHB) production can be achieved primarily by promoting ketosis. Here are some methods to stimulate the production of BHB:

1. Dietary Ketosis:

- Ketogenic Diet: Adopt a high-fat, moderate-protein, and low-carbohydrate diet. This restricts glucose availability, prompting the body to produce ketones, including BHB.

- Fasting: Intermittent fasting or prolonged fasting can push the body into ketosis as it depletes liver glycogen stores, leading to increased BHB production.

2. Exercise:

- Prolonged physical activity, especially aerobic exercise, can deplete glycogen stores and stimulate BHB production.

3. MCT Oil: Consuming medium-chain triglyceride (MCT) oil can increase ketone production since MCTs are rapidly absorbed and converted into ketones in the liver.

4. Exogenous Ketones: Directly consuming BHB salts or esters will raise BHB levels in the blood. These are often found in ketone supplements.

5. Limiting Protein: While the ketogenic diet is moderate in protein, consuming too much protein can inhibit ketosis. The amino acids from excess protein can be converted to glucose through gluconeogenesis, reducing BHB production.

6. Alcohol Abstinence: Alcohol can inhibit fat metabolism in the liver, which can interfere with ketone production.

7. Proper Sleep: Sleep disturbances can affect ketone production, so ensuring adequate and quality sleep can support higher BHB levels.

8. Manage Stress: Chronic stress can elevate cortisol levels, increasing blood sugar and potentially reducing BHB production.

Remember, before making significant changes to your diet or lifestyle, especially if considering fasting or supplements, it's essential to consult with a healthcare professional to ensure safety and appropriateness for your individual situation.

Chapter 10
Menopause and Mindful Fasting

Ketones, the energy-packed molecules that act as alternative fuel for our bodies, can be attained in several noteworthy ways. First up, there's the ketogenic diet mentioned in Chapter 8. By significantly cutting down on carbohydrates, the body enters a state called ketosis, which primarily burns fats, producing ketones. The second avenue? Fasting. When you abstain from food, your body exhausts its glucose reserves and relies on ketones for energy. For the ladies navigating the choppy waters of menopause, fasting might just be the lighthouse they've been searching for. Beyond ketone production, fasting offers potential benefits like hormonal balance, reduced hot flashes, improved sleep, and enhanced mood. It's like giving your body a well-deserved break and potentially easing those menopausal speed bumps.

In this chapter, we will delve into the physiology of fasting, and its implications for weight gain and obesity. We will also examine the potential advantages fasting offers your health.

Hormonal Harmony vs. Caloric Calculations: Dissecting the Two Titans of Weight Gain Theories

The fundamental question at the heart of this discussion revolves around the two predominant models of weight gain: the calorie model and the hormonal model, which we touched on in Chapter 6. The calorie model posits that all you need to understand about weight gain is measuring food energy in calories. It suggests that a calorie is a calorie; thus, all calories are equally fattening. This concept has been the cornerstone of much of the dietary advice we've received. Even recent guidelines from 2021 emphasise the importance of adjusting energy intake and expenditure, essentially advocating the age-old advice of "eating less and moving more." This advice assumes that weight gain is entirely within your control, solely on calorie management.

However, there exists another perspective known as the hormonal model, which takes a more comprehensive approach. While acknowledging that food contains energy, it also believes that what we eat triggers different hormonal responses. For instance, consuming cookies will cause a significant surge in insulin and blood glucose levels. At the same time, a meal of salmon or an egg with minimal carbohydrates won't elicit the same response. These hormonal reactions serve as instructions for our bodies, guiding various metabolic processes. In 2021, prominent researchers, including David Ludwig and Walter Willett from Harvard, proposed the carbohydrate-insulin model, highlighting the central role of insulin as a key hormone. Insulin primarily functions as a storage hormone, promoting glycogen and body fat synthesis while inhibiting their breakdown. Thus, this model underscores the importance of considering both calorie quantity and the quality of calories, as they induce different hormonal responses.

The cornerstone of this discussion is the energy balance equation, which asserts that body fat is a product of calories in and calories out. This equation is frequently cited in discussions advocating for caloric deficits to lose weight. However, it's crucial to understand that a true caloric deficit never occurs in this equation. It's always a balanced equation. The other two must adjust to maintain equilibrium when you alter one component. Hence, claims that simply eating fewer calories will lead to weight loss oversimplify the complex interplay of factors. Merely reducing calorie intake doesn't guarantee fat loss, as it doesn't account for the potential decrease in metabolic rate. If you consume fewer calories, your body may adapt by burning fewer calories, potentially keeping your body fat unchanged. This phenomenon aligns with the laws of thermodynamics and challenges the oversimplified notion that "eating less equals losing weight." The real-world question becomes whether reducing calorie intake results in fat loss or whether your metabolic rate decreases.

The Metabolic Response to Calorie Reduction

In 1944, Dr. Ancel Keys conducted a landmark study called "The Biology of Human Starvation." This study I covered in Chapter 5 was prompted by the need to understand the physiological effects of insufficient food during World War II. Subjects in the study were placed on a reduced calorie intake, specifically consuming 1570 calories per day. This calorie restriction was primarily based on starchy, low-protein, and low-fat foods, reflecting the limited dietary options in war-torn Europe.

The diet composition, which included low-fat foods and approximately 1500 calories, may seem somewhat similar to dietary advice given today. However, the results of this study shed light on how the human body responds to calorie reduction. Researchers found that the participants' metabolic rates decreased significantly by approximately 40 per cent. Various physiological changes occurred; their heart volume decreased, overall strength diminished, and heart rates slowed. These participants also experienced a drop in body temperature, leading to feelings of coldness, fatigue, and overall discomfort. This discomfort arose from the body's inability to receive sufficient energy to support the functioning of vital organs, such as the heart, liver, and brain, which generate body heat. This study highlighted that when calorie intake is reduced, the body naturally responds by lowering its calorie expenditure to maintain equilibrium.

It's important to note that the body's adaptability is a fundamental aspect of homeostasis. If you reduce your daily calorie intake by 500 calories, for example, you might expect to lose about a pound per week. However, this does not imply that you would continue losing weight indefinitely until reaching zero. In reality, the body adapts to the reduced calorie intake almost immediately.

Adaptive Metabolism: The Interplay of Caloric Intake and Energy Expenditure

In 1971, a study conducted an experiment similar to Dr. Ancel Keys' earlier work, investigating the effects of underfeeding on subjects. The findings revealed a consistent pattern: when individuals are underfed, their metabolic rates tend to decrease by approximately 10 to 20 per cent. This phenomenon has been observed repeatedly in various studies over the years.

One prominent example illustrating this concept comes from "The Biggest Loser," an American reality series focused on weight loss competition. This show's participants followed calorie-restricted diets to shed excess pounds. Their experiences showed that as they lost weight, their metabolic rates continued to decline. Despite their attempts to compensate for this decreasing metabolic rate through increased physical activity, there came a point where they couldn't sustain such high levels of exercise. Importantly, it's crucial to understand that exercise predominantly affects skeletal muscle and has a limited impact on the metabolic rates of vital organs like the liver, lungs, and kidneys. In response to reduced calorie intake, these internal organs adapt by decreasing their metabolic rates to preserve energy balance.

Indeed, this decline in metabolic rate with calorie reduction has been extensively documented. In 1991, a meta-analysis of 29 studies delved into the relationship between caloric restriction and changes in resting metabolic rate (often referred to as "calories out"). The consensus among these studies was striking: nearly all reported a decrease in metabolic rates ranging from 10 to 20 percent when calorie intake was reduced. This collective body of evidence firmly establishes that a decrease in energy expenditure is a consistent response to energy restriction. In simpler terms, if you eat less, your body will naturally burn fewer calories, potentially leading to minimal changes in body fat.

In clinical practice, the observations align closely with what scientific research has revealed about the interplay of calorie balance, exercise, and weight management. When we consider the first law of thermodynamics, which emphasises that there are three variables – calories in, calories out, and body fat – we can explore how changes in one or more of these factors impact our body composition.

Firstly, let's examine the scenario of increasing exercise to lose weight. While exercise is essential for overall health and fitness, it may not be a panacea for weight loss. Increasing physical activity primarily affects calories out, but it also has an unexpected twist. Researchers at Harvard conducted a meta-analysis in 2021, examining the effects of exercise training interventions on energy intake. Although they initially included 48 studies, the analysis eventually focused on high-quality studies due to varying research quality. The consensus from these high-quality studies was clear: when you exercise, you tend to experience an increase in hunger. This heightened appetite can naturally lead to an increase in calorie consumption.

Consider a practical example: during acute exercise, such as a soccer game, your appetite might temporarily decrease because you're pre-occupied. However, once you've finished exercising, hunger tends to kick in, often leading to increased calorie intake.

Now, let's delve into the "energy gap" concept associated with different activities. You're either in a positive or negative energy balance when you engage in activities, whether it's mild exercise or even watching TV. For instance, watching TV typically results in a positive energy balance, meaning you're consuming more calories than you're expending – about 100 calories per hour. Surprisingly, while beneficial for overall health, mild exercise doesn't necessarily lead to a negative energy balance and weight loss. In fact, it also results in a positive energy balance of approximately 99 calories per hour. This phenomenon can be attributed to the increased hunger that accompanies exercise.

You typically need to engage in more intense physical activities to achieve a neutral or negative caloric balance through exercise. At this level of intensity, you might finally expend more calories than you consume, contributing to potential weight loss.

In summary, the advice to "do a little bit of exercise" is undoubtedly valuable for overall health and well-being. Still, it may not be the most effective strategy for significant weight loss. Importantly, these observations don't violate the laws of thermodynamics; they simply underscore the complex interplay between calorie balance, exercise, and appetite regulation.

Run More, Burn Less? The Metabolic Mischief Behind Caloric Math

When we consider calorie expenditure, it's not solely about exercise; your resting metabolic rate also plays a significant role. Calorie expenditure consists of two primary components: the calories burned through physical activity, including exercise, and the calories expended at rest, which is your metabolic rate. Increasing exercise can make you hungrier, but another intriguing aspect to consider is the potential decrease in your resting metabolic rate to compensate for increased activity.

Two theoretical models help us understand this phenomenon. The "additive" model suggests that your baseline metabolic rate remains constant, and exercise simply adds to the total calorie expenditure. In this model, the more exercise you do, the more energy you burn, leading to weight loss. On the other hand, the "constrained" model proposes that at a certain point, additional exercise will be met with a decrease in your resting metabolic rate to maintain energy balance. This raises the question: which model accurately reflects reality?

Research conducted in 2016 shed light on this matter. Using doubly labelled water, scientists studied 332 adults across five populations to investigate the relationship between increased physical activity and total energy expenditure. What they discovered supported the constrained model. Beyond a certain threshold of increased physical activity, there was no further significant increase in total energy expenditure. In other words, the additional calories burned through exercise were matched by decreased resting metabolic rate. This finding emphasises the principle of homeostasis, a fundamental aspect of life where the body strives to maintain balance.

Returning to "The Biggest Loser" study from 2021, participants followed a calorie-restricted diet while increasing exercise. As we know, their metabolic rates decreased. Researchers examined how the amount of exercise correlated with changes in metabolic rate. Surprisingly, they found that those who engaged in more exercise experienced a greater decrease in metabolic rate. This phenomenon can be attributed to your internal organs, such as the heart, lungs, kidneys, and brain, collectively using less energy. Even though skeletal muscle activity increased with more exercise, this increase was matched by a decrease in energy generation by vital organs. Therefore, there's a point where additional exercise doesn't yield a net benefit in terms of calorie expenditure.

In summary, the interaction between exercise, calorie expenditure, and metabolic rate is intricate. While exercise is essential for health and well-being, there's a point at which increased physical activity may be offset by a decrease in resting metabolic rate, reinforcing the body's inclination toward balance and adaptation.

Hormonal Hijinks: Why Counting Calories is Only Half the Weighty Tale

The concept that weight management isn't solely governed by the number of calories consumed versus calories burned has led to a more profound understanding of how hormones play a pivotal role in this process. Hormones are the body's messengers, orchestrating various metabolic functions, and ultimately, they dictate whether your body will store or burn energy. The idea is applicable not only to eating but also to exercise. Hormones hold the reins in our body's intricate metabolic symphony.

One hormone that plays a central role in this narrative is insulin. It functions as a nutrient sensor, signalling to your body that food is available and prompting it to store energy. When insulin levels are high, you enter a state of fat storage, as insulin inhibits lipolysis, the breakdown of stored fat. This inhibition occurs logically because insulin signals your body to store incoming energy, not utilise reserves simultaneously.

On the contrary, when insulin levels drop, which can occur during fasting or periods of reduced calorie intake, a cascade of counter-regulatory hormones comes into play. These hormones, including noradrenaline, growth hormone, and cortisol, signal your body to release stored energy into the bloodstream. Your body shifts from storage to utilisation mode, which is crucial for maintaining energy balance, especially during fasting or low-calorie periods.

Consider two scenarios to illustrate the significance of hormonal influence. In the first scenario, you maintain high insulin levels throughout the day by consuming frequent low-fat, high-carbohydrate meals. Let's say you were expending 2000 calories daily. Now, if you reduce your calorie intake to 1500 calories while keeping your insulin levels high, your body's options for energy are limited. You can't readily tap into fat stores due to the ongoing insulin signal to store energy. Consequently, your body is left to lower its metabolic rate to maintain equilibrium, as it can't access fat reserves efficiently.

In the second scenario, you consume 1500 calories but employ intermittent fasting. During fasting, insulin levels drop, permitting the breakdown of fat and glycogen stores for energy. In this case, despite the reduced calorie intake, your body can access stored energy efficiently, maintaining energy balance without significantly lowering metabolic rate.

Both scenarios adhere to the laws of thermodynamics, keeping the energy equation balanced. However, they illustrate hormones' critical role in determining how your body handles calorie intake and expenditure.

The pivotal question arises: which model holds more power in understanding weight regulation, the traditional calorie in, calorie out model or the hormonal model of obesity? An intriguing study conducted a few years ago provides valuable insights. Researchers deliberately kept insulin levels high while reducing calorie intake. According to the conventional calorie-based model, one might expect weight loss due to reduced calories. However, when viewed through the lens of the hormonal model, high insulin levels could drive weight gain, as hormones hold significant sway over our body's responses.

This study underscores the significance of hormonal influence and invites a more nuanced understanding of weight regulation that extends beyond simple calorie counting.

Beyond Calories: The Crucial Role of Insulin in Weight Management

In a pivotal study conducted in 1993 by Henry and colleagues, the focus was on individuals with type 2 diabetes. Over a six-month period, researchers administered varying amounts of insulin, gradually increasing it to a substantial 100 units per day. Simultaneously, calorie intake was reduced from approximately 2000 calories to 1700 calories daily, resulting in a daily deficit of 300 calories. According to the traditional calorie in, calorie out model, this should have led to significant weight loss.

However, the results were far from expected. Rather than shedding pounds, the subjects gained 20 pounds during this period, despite the calorie deficit. This perplexing outcome underscores the notion that perhaps it was never just about calories. Instead, it appears that insulin, the hormone responsible for signalling your body to store calories as fat, played a significant role. As a result, the rest of the body had less energy to burn, and this dynamic explains how weight gain can occur even when consuming fewer calories.

In the broader context, calories and hormones are vital factors in weight management's intricate dance. Ignoring either aspect is an oversimplification. Insulin, in particular, takes centre stage in this narrative. Intermittent fasting emerges as a powerful strategy for reducing insulin levels, as during fasting, you're essentially consuming zero calories, resulting in the lowest possible insulin levels. Low-carbohydrate diets also play a role by stimulating insulin to a lesser extent, although they don't quite match the effectiveness of fasting. Regardless of the approach chosen, understanding the interplay between hormones and calories is key.

It's essential to avoid the trap of thinking, "I'll fast and then eat whatever I want." While fasting addresses the hormone aspect, calorie control remains crucial because energy intake is still a factor. To achieve optimal weight loss, managing hormones and calories effectively is necessary.

Clocking In on Calorie Curfews: Why This Study Might Need a Time-Out

You may have seen a New York Times headline in 2022 declaring, "Scientists Find No Benefit to Time-Restricted Eating". This was drawn from a recent study published in the New England Journal of Medicine in 2022. Researchers investigated calorie-restricted diets with or without time-restricted eating, which involves intermittent fasting. At the one-year mark, there was no statistically significant difference in weight loss between the two groups, suggesting that perhaps calorie restriction alone was sufficient. However, a closer look reveals an interesting pattern. At six months, a small difference of 0.5 kg emerged, and this difference grew to 1.8 kg by the one-year mark. While not statistically significant, this divergence prompts further inquiry.

One must consider that the study might be underpowered to detect a significant difference. When investigating the impact of fasting, the subjects increased their fasting duration from 13.8 hours to 16 hours, a shift of less than three hours. This underlines the importance of not jumping to hasty conclusions.

The study's conclusion, stating that there are no benefits to time-restricted eating, warrants scrutiny. The 28% increase in weight loss may not be statistically significant, but clinically, such a difference could have substantial long-term implications for metabolic health.

Additionally, the study's design posed limitations. Comparing two correlated variables, such as calorie restriction and time-restricted eating, requires nuanced analysis. Simply measuring the outcomes while holding one variable constant doesn't negate the benefits of the variable being studied. This is akin to assessing a weight loss drug: if the drug helps you consume fewer calories and lose weight, concluding that it's a beneficial drug is valid. However, demonstrating the same weight loss with fixed calorie intake doesn't negate the drug's benefits. The key benefit is that the drug facilitates calorie reduction more effectively.

Similarly, in the study of calorie restriction and time-restricted eating, if time-restricted eating enables individuals to eat fewer calories, that remains a significant advantage. Thus, it's crucial to consider the nuances and potential benefits of both calorie control and hormone regulation in achieving effective weight management. When evaluating studies and news headlines, it's crucial to scrutinise the research methodology rather than being swayed by attention-grabbing headlines alone.

Time-Restricted Eating: A Natural Calorie Reduction

Numerous studies highlight the positive effects of time-restricted eating on calorie intake. In a study in the journal Cell Metabolism, participants were divided into groups with four- or six-hour time-restricted eating windows. In contrast, a control group had unrestricted eating hours. The fascinating outcome was that, even without explicit instructions to reduce calorie consumption, those practising time-restricted eating naturally consumed about 500 fewer calories daily. This calorie reduction occurred without individuals consciously monitoring their calorie intake. The logic is straightforward: when you limit the time available for eating, it becomes easier to consume fewer calories. For instance, if you establish a rule of not eating after 6 p.m., late-night snacking temptations are mitigated as they fall outside your eating window.

Emotional eating, a common culprit behind excessive calorie consumption and weight gain, should not be dismissed as irrelevant. It often serves as the root cause of overeating, making it essential to address this emotional component to achieve sustained weight loss success. Identifying why you are gaining weight is crucial. If excessive calorie intake is the issue, delve deeper into why you are consuming too many calories. In some cases, the problem may stem from having too many opportunities to eat throughout the day. In such instances, restricting your eating window can significantly boost your weight loss efforts.

Consider a scenario where you're consuming 2,000 calories daily and burning the same amount. You follow a traditional breakfast, lunch, and dinner routine. Time-restricted eating doesn't aim to increase or decrease calorie intake but instead focuses on shifting meal timing. By doing so, you provide your body with a fasting period during which insulin levels drop, allowing for the utilisation of energy from fat stores.

Body fat essentially represents stored calories from past meals. However, if insulin levels remain elevated, these energy stores remain inaccessible. The only way to access this stored energy is to eat more, meeting your energy requirements through additional calories.

Individuals with conditions like type 2 diabetes, characterised by insulin resistance and excessive insulin production, face a particularly challenging scenario. A significant portion is swiftly redirected to fat stores when they consume calories due to high insulin levels. Consequently, their bodies signal hunger even when ample energy reserves exist within their fat stores.

For those on low-fat diets, consuming high-carb, low-fat meals like white bread with jam can trigger sharp spikes in blood glucose and insulin levels. This results in the rapid storage of breakfast calories as fat, leaving little to burn as energy stores remain locked. Mid-morning cravings become inevitable as the body clamours for additional sustenance. However, eating a breakfast like bacon and eggs, which leads to lower insulin spikes, can sustain feelings of fullness and reduce mid-morning hunger.

The takeaway is that energy and hormones play pivotal roles in weight management. Ignoring one in favour of the other oversimplifies the complex processes involved.

Critics who advocate the calorie-restricted model often espouse the idea that weight control is solely within conscious control. They assert,

"Just eat less and exercise more," implying that being overweight is exclusively an individual's responsibility due to overeating and insufficient physical activity. But is it really that simple?

Hunger Games: Why Are You Hungry All The Time?

Beyond the surface, exploring the underlying factors contributing to overeating is crucial. Perhaps you are constantly hungry, a sensation driven by various hormones regulating appetite. Ghrelin, often called the hunger hormone, and GLP-1, the satiety hormone, play significant roles. When you feel full, you naturally eat less, and vice versa. Additionally, adrenaline influences your sympathetic tone and your metabolic rate. A higher metabolic rate leads to increased energy expenditure.

Then there's insulin, a hormone long associated with weight gain. A telling example comes from the DCCT trial in 2001, where type 1 diabetics were administered varying insulin doses. Predictably, those receiving higher insulin doses achieved better glucose control, but nearly 30 per cent experienced significant weight gain during the trial. The correlation between insulin and weight gain is a common observation among patients prescribed insulin, many of whom report substantial weight increases.

Insulin functions as a hormonal agent, similar to GLP-1. In a trial published in the New England Journal of Medicine in 2021, participants who received weekly semaglutide injections, a GLP-1 agonist, exhibited a remarkable 15% reduction in body weight over 68 weeks.

Interestingly, one of the side effects of semaglutide is nausea, which contributes to appetite reduction. When individuals abstain from eating due to nausea, they naturally shed pounds, partly because this decrease in food consumption also leads to reduced insulin production.

Nicotine, commonly found in cigarettes, is another hormonal agent that affects multiple facets of weight regulation. Smokers tend to have lower body weights than non-smokers, attributed to nicotine's sympathomimetic properties, which elevate noradrenaline and norepinephrine levels, thereby increasing metabolic rates. Simultaneously, nicotine impacts GABA receptors, diminishing appetite while enhancing feelings of satiety. Consequently, smokers often experience reduced hunger and increased calorie expenditure. However, when they quit smoking, the lost weight tends to return.

This complex interplay of hormones highlights that weight management goes far beyond calorie counting and exercise. Understanding the hormonal drivers of hunger and metabolism is paramount to achieving lasting results.

The Fasting Secret: How Skipping Meals Can Make You Less Hungry and Boost Your Fat-Burning Furnace

Understanding how fasting affects hunger and metabolic rate provides valuable insights into its effectiveness as a weight management tool. Ghrelin, the hunger hormone, can serve as a key indicator of these effects. In a study involving 24-hour fasting, researchers observed the typical ghrelin spikes corresponding to breakfast, lunch, and dinner. Intriguingly, skipping a meal, such as lunch, led to a temporary increase in hunger, but ghrelin levels quickly returned to baseline. This phenomenon also occurred when dinner was skipped. Over several days of fasting, ghrelin fluctuations aligned with habitual eating patterns, but after a few days, ghrelin levels began to decline. This mirrors the experience of many who fast for extended periods, as hunger tends to diminish over time.

Comparing caloric restriction to alternate daily fasting in another study revealed distinct differences in ghrelin response—caloric restriction led to an increase in ghrelin levels, indicating heightened hunger. In contrast, alternate daily fasting did not produce the same surge in ghrelin. This suggests that fasting methods may better regulate appetite compared to traditional calorie restriction.

Contrary to the misconception that fasting dampens metabolic rate, research shows the opposite effect. When subjects fasted for four days, their calorie expenditure increased by approximately 10 percent on the fourth day compared to day zero. This metabolic boost is attributed to elevated sympathetic tone, marked by increased adrenaline and growth hormone levels. Growth hormone helps preserve lean muscle mass, contributing to a higher resting energy expenditure.

A study conducted in 2002, which examined human adipose tissue after 72 hours of fasting, reinforced this finding. Researchers observed a rise in noradrenaline levels alongside a notable increase in resting energy expenditure from 1684 to 1729 calories after three days of fasting. These results demonstrate that subjects burned more energy on day three than on the initial day.

Dispelling the myth of fasting lowering metabolic rate, these findings emphasise the hormonal benefits of fasting, including reduced hunger and increased metabolic activity. While calorie restriction often leads to decreased metabolic rates and heightened hunger, fasting appears to offer a more favourable balance, making it a promising approach for sustainable weight loss.

Unlocking the Doctor's Weight Loss Secret: Intermittent Fasting Demystified

Have you ever wondered how doctors maintain their weight or even shed those extra pounds when needed? A fascinating study of 900 female doctors provides surprising insights into their go-to weight loss strategy. These physicians, while not grossly overweight, successfully shed an average of 13.2 pounds. The real revelation? A whopping 75 per cent of them credited intermittent fasting for their results.

But here's the kicker—only 25-30 per cent of these medical professionals recommend this method to their patients. A puzzling discrepancy piqued my curiosity and led me to write this book. Everyone deserves access to the latest scientific findings, empowering them to make informed health and weight management choices.

Let's address a common concern: does intermittent fasting leave you vulnerable to eating disorders? Many worry that fasting might disrupt tryptophan, a precursor for serotonin, potentially leading to mild depression and increased susceptibility to eating disorders.

However, multiple studies have delved into this issue, providing reassuring results. In a study assessing 218 participants over a 24-hour fast, researchers found that fasting did not significantly predict an increase in eating disorders. Similarly, in a 2002 trial involving individuals with diagnosed eating disorders, subjecting them to fasting did not trigger eating pathology.

Fasting can be an efficient way to regulate calorie intake and promote fat burning. This is because it gradually reduces hunger over time and paradoxically boosts metabolic rates, opposing conventional wisdom. While some sources may claim that time-restricted eating offers no benefits, it's quite the opposite.

The Power of Structure: How Intermittent Fasting Simplifies Weight Management

It's no secret that managing your weight can be a challenge. But what if there were a simple, science-backed approach that could make the journey smoother? Intermittent fasting offers structured eating windows that require no calorie counting. This innovative strategy empowers you to reduce calorie intake, all while building healthy habits effortlessly.

You create a clear eating schedule with time-restricted eating, eliminating the guesswork. This method is straightforward, unlike calorie counting, which can be confusing and time-consuming. It's not about what you eat but when you eat, making it easy to adopt. Whether you're a seasoned pro or new to weight management, this approach can work for you.

Fasting: A Universal Solution for Weight Management

In a world where diets can be complicated, expensive, and time-consuming, fasting stands out as a free, convenient, and flexible alternative. It doesn't require unique meal plans or expensive organic ingredients. Fasting can save you time, as you'll spend less on groceries and skip the lengthy meal preparation.

Perhaps one of its most significant advantages is its flexibility. You're not tied to fasting daily; you can adapt it to your schedule. Holidays are coming up? Take a break and resume fasting afterwards. It's a strategy that can seamlessly fit into any lifestyle, offering a universal solution to weight management.

Chapter 11
Unlocking the Mysteries of Fasting

Fasting, a practice as old as time itself, can be divided into five remarkable stages, as deciphered by the pioneering work of Dr. George Cahill, a luminary in the field of medicine at Harvard Medical School. These stages offer a profound insight into how our bodies adapt during food scarcity and where they source their glucose for energy.

To comprehend these stages, it's vital to grasp that our bodies predominantly rely on two sources of fuel: glucose, derived from carbohydrates, and fat, stored in the form of triglycerides within adipocytes, our fat cells. Most cells in our body, with a few exceptions like the brain, are versatile and can harness glucose or triglycerides to meet their energy needs, akin to a hybrid car that can switch between gasoline and electricity.

Let's delve into the five stages of fasting and understand what transpires within our bodies during each phase:

Stage One: The Feeding Stage (0-4 Hours After a Meal)

At the outset of a meal, glucose is abundant in the bloodstream, thanks to a mixture of carbohydrates, proteins, and fats. Nutrient sensors like insulin and mTOR signal the body to store this surplus energy for later use. Glucose is stored as glycogen in the liver, and triglycerides are sequestered in fat cells.

Stage Two: The Post-Absorptive Stage (4-16 Hours)

Insulin and mTOR levels gradually decline as the hours pass after a meal. Most cells continue to rely on glucose, but now it primarily comes from glycogen stored in the liver. Without dietary glucose, the body may use ketones as an alternative energy source. This stage is pivotal for reducing the risk of insulin-related diseases and initiating salt and water release, lowering blood pressure and reducing bloating.

Stage Three: Gluconeogenesis (16-30 Hours)

Glycogen reserves in the liver begin to deplete during this phase. The body turns to gluconeogenesis, producing glucose primarily from protein sources. Gluconeogenesis may stimulate autophagy, a process of cellular rejuvenation and self-regeneration. This phase ensures that the body efficiently uses amino acids and discards unnecessary proteins, like excess skin.

Stage Four: Ketosis (>2 Days)

Beyond the 48-hour mark, the body enters ketosis, where the liver converts triglycerides into ketones. Ketones are a significant energy source, especially for the brain, improving mental clarity and performance. Ketosis is considered an efficient state for brain function and has applications in treating epilepsy.

Stage Five: Protein Conservation (6-7 Days and Beyond)

In this stage, the body relies primarily on stored body fat for energy. Gluconeogenesis still contributes minimally to energy needs, while the bulk comes from fat. Hunger signals, including the hunger hormone ghrelin, significantly decrease as the body feeds off its own fat stores.

These five stages elucidate the remarkable adaptability of the human body during fasting. While fasting may not suit everyone, it provides valuable insights into our metabolic processes and the potential health benefits of controlled fasting periods. Whether it's for a few days or intermittent fasting, understanding these stages can inform your approach to this age-old practice, promoting better health and well-being.

Real-Life Success Stories and Total Transformation

When my patients come to see me, we discuss their health goals and aspirations. While fasting isn't exclusively for those battling weight issues or health concerns, it's crucial to understand your objectives and find a sustainable approach that doesn't isolate you from your social circle. Life is a delicate balance, and it's best lived in moderation.

However, I can attest that fasting has proven remarkably effective for some of my patients. Take Linda (whose name has been changed to respect her privacy), for instance. At 59 years old, Linda found herself carrying excess weight, leading to a concerning emergency room visit. Her doctor suggested surgery as an option, but Linda courageously declined. Instead, she decided to take her health into her own hands, which changed her life. Excess weight had triggered a cascade of health issues, from diabetes to high blood pressure and even lower back pain.

When Linda and I first met, we both understood the urgency of her situation. We decided on a 5:2 fasting schedule, where she would fast for two days a week and eat normally for the remaining five days. This fasting regimen primarily involved water, with a hint of coffee and green tea. Linda also took the initiative to become more physically active, incorporating brisk walks into her routine at least three hours a week.

Remarkably, by the fourth week, Linda took things a step further. She engaged a personal trainer and began two hours of resistance training each week. She harnessed the boost in growth hormone production that fasting provides. In just three months, Linda's transformation was nothing short of astonishing. She shed over 20 kilograms and achieved her goal of a healthy waist-to-hip ratio. But it wasn't merely about weight loss but a holistic transformation. Linda, a menopausal woman who initially struggled with climbing a single flight of stairs, now revels in 5-kilometre hikes across challenging terrain.

Stories like Linda's drive my passion to educate as many people as possible. I hope that others can experience similar life-changing benefits by sharing this knowledge. While medicine has undoubtedly brought immense benefits to the world, the solution doesn't always reside in a pill. You can take control of your health and embark on a journey of self-transformation, enhancing not only your body but your entire life.

Chapter 12
Muscle Magic

Resistance training, often also referred to as strength or weight training, is a form of exercise that improves muscular strength and endurance. When you hear "resistance," think "opposition" – it involves causing the muscles to contract against an external force. The goal is to build the strength and size of skeletal muscles gradually.

The American College of Sports Medicine (ACSM) recommends adults engage in resistance training at least twice weekly to promote musculoskeletal health. However, a study by Kruger et al. revealed only 20% of women adhere to this guideline, falling short of the Healthy People 2020 target of 24%. The study further indicated men participate approximately 30% more in resistance training than women.

Resistance training, defined by the ACSM, enhances muscular fitness by exercising against external resistance. Popular methods include free weights, weight machines, resistance bands, and body weight exercises. It's crucial for preserving lean muscle mass for daily functions and sporting activities. This significance is underscored by the natural decline of muscle mass with age, which is associated with various medical conditions and reduced quality of life.

Surprisingly, despite the proven benefits, research indicates that women engage less in resistance training than men. The benefits span improved muscle strength, body composition, metabolic efficiency, and bone density. Beyond physical health, regular resistance training is linked to psychological benefits.

Muscle's Hidden Metabolism: Setting the Scene

During menopause, the body undergoes a myriad of changes. For many, the focus often zeroes in on hormones, hot flashes, and bones. But there's a hero in this narrative that usually takes the backseat – our muscles. More than just powerhouses of strength, muscles play an intricate role in metabolic regulation. The question has been brewing in the medical world: Can resistance muscle training offer relief from menopausal symptoms?

With menopause, the decline in oestrogen levels can lead to loss of bone density, increased fat accumulation, muscle mass reduction, and other physical changes. Resistance training serves as a countermeasure to these challenges.

Assessing the Impact of Resistance Training on Post-menopausal Women: Insights from a 2023 Study

A study was done in 2023 to assess the effects of resistance muscle training for postmenopausal women. At the heart of this exploration was a simple yet profound aim: To gauge the potential pros and cons of resistance muscle training for postmenopausal women.

With the objective clear, the researchers initiated a deep dive into existing research. Databases like MEDLINE, EMBASE, CENTRAL, PEDro, LILACS, and SPORTDiscus, some of the most reputed in the field, were scoured up until December 2021. From the vast literature, twelve randomised clinical trials stood out, encapsulating the experiences of 452 participants. Here's the intriguing part:

Compared to no exercise, resistance training (spanning up to 16 weeks) showcased an enhanced functional capacity, improved bone mineral density, a noticeable reduction in the frequency of hot flashes and a decrease in fat mass. Pitting resistance training against aerobic exercises revealed a more pronounced reduction in hot flash frequency and fat mass with resistance training. However, quality of life and body mass index remained unaffected.

Unveiling the Power of Strength Training for Women

While many associate resistance training with the male fitness sphere, the myriad benefits it offers women are undeniable and vast.

1. Bolstering Bone Density – As women journey through life, bone density wanes, notably post-menopause. Resistance training judiciously stresses bones, enhancing their strength. Since osteoporosis plagues 10 million Americans—with women at heightened risk—it's crucial for them to prioritise bone health as they advance in years.

2. Muscle Mass Augmentation – Muscles underpin every human motion. As such, preserving them safeguards against injuries and enhances daily tasks' ease, from mundane stair-climbing to more demanding ones. And for those women wary of acquiring a "masculine" physique, fret not: weightlifting refines rather than bulks the body, promoting muscle growth and honing the overall physique.

3. An Ally in Weight Management – Dismantling prevalent myths, resistance training is an effective weight-loss strategy. It burns calories akin to cardio exercises and fuels Excess Post-Oxygen Consumption (EPOC). In this phenomenon, the body continues its caloric combustion long after the workout.

4. Serenading Sound Sleep – Emerging research attests to the enhanced sleep quality enjoyed by women who resistance train. Such

restorative sleep is a linchpin for holistic well-being, especially as the years roll on.

5. Energizing the Everyday – While exercise invariably triggers mood-elevating endorphins, prolonged cardio can sap energy reserves. Conversely, strength training sessions, often spanning 30 to 60 minutes, invigorate, ensuring a spirited day ahead.

6. Functional Strength for Daily Hustles – Women's days are action-packed, from navigating demanding office hours to tending to toddlers or managing household chores. Strength training ensures they have the requisite stamina and strength, fortifying core regions like the back, legs, and upper body.

7. Shielding the Heart – With heart disease touted as the primary femme fatale, consistent exercise is a crucial preventive measure with bi-weekly strength training sessions that can significantly uplift heart health.

8. Mitigating Stress – Though cardio's stress-alleviating prowess is well-documented, strength training too, emerges as a potent stress buster. This becomes even more pertinent because women are predisposed to manifesting physical stress symptoms, such as migraines or gastrointestinal upsets. Beyond mental tranquillity, this also fortifies overall health.

9. Confidence Resurgence – In a world awash with media-dictated female body ideals, the goal-centric approach of strength training offers a refreshing change. Shifting from aesthetics to functionality—like enhancing speed or lifting capacity—strength training has been linked to enhanced body perception among women. As an added boon, the aesthetic transformations naturally follow, even if they aren't the primary aim.

Strength training isn't merely a fitness routine—it's an empowering lifestyle choice for women, promising both physical vitality and psychological well-being.

Tailored Exercises for Menopausal Women

1. Dumbbell Exercises:
    - Bicep Curls: Targets the biceps.
    - Shoulder Press: Focuses on the shoulders.
    - Tricep Extension: Aims at the triceps.
  2. Bodyweight Exercises:
    - Squats: Engages the thighs, buttocks, and lower back.
    - Lunges: Works the thighs and buttocks.
    - Push-ups: (modified versions if needed) Strengthens the chest, shoulders, and arms.
  3. Resistance Band Workouts:
    - Band Pull-apart: Targets the rear shoulder muscles.
    - Seated Rows: Strengthens the middle back.
    - Leg Presses: Using a band; it works on the leg muscles.
  4. Machines at the Gym (if available and accessible):
    - Leg Press Machine: Targets the leg muscles.
    - Chest Press Machine: Focuses on the chest and tricep muscles.
    - Lat Pulldown Machine: Strengthens the upper back.
  5. Functional Training:
    - Step-ups:* Using a bench or step, this exercise is excellent for leg strength and balance.
    - Planks: Engages the core, strengthening the midsection.

Crafting a Routine

For optimal results, menopausal women should aim for 2-3 days of resistance training each week. Here's a sample beginner's routine:

1. Warm up with a 10-minute brisk walk.

2. Choose 5-6 exercises, focusing on major muscle groups.

3. Start with one set of each exercise, performing 10-12 repetitions.

4. As strength and endurance improve, gradually increase to 2-3 sets.

Safety First

As beneficial as resistance training is, it's essential to ensure safety:

1. Form is Key: Proper technique prevents injuries.

2. Progress Slowly: Begin with lighter weights and increase gradually.

3. Rest and Recovery: Allow a day's rest between sessions to let muscles recover.

4. Consultation: Before starting any resistance training regimen, it's wise to consult with a healthcare provider, especially if there are underlying health conditions or concerns.

Resistance training is a versatile tool that can be tailored to the needs and abilities of menopausal women. Not only does it combat physiological changes associated with menopause, but it also empowers women to lead active, strong, and healthy lives in their post-menopausal years.

Chapter 13
Cracking the Code of Metabolic Health

When I think about metabolic health, I remember a remarkable encounter with a 71-year-old woman. This wise woman had transformed her health in her later years, defying the stereotypes associated with ageing. Her story was a testament to the incredible power of exercise and a healthy lifestyle. She had once been obese, hypertensive, a social smoker, and lived a sedentary life well into her early 50s. But one day, she decided to make a change. She took up writing, jogging, and pondering the mysteries of life. Over the next three decades, she transformed herself into a model of vitality. At 71, her metabolic health resembled that of a healthy person in their 30s – an astounding achievement. It's a powerful example of how exercise can shape our longevity and well-being.

Zone 2 Training for Menopausal Marvels: Heartbeats, Hormones, and Healing

As menopause sets in, women often confront a myriad of physical and emotional changes, some of which can be both challenging and frustrating. However, the ever-evolving field of exercise physiology offers a silver lining: Zone 2 training. But what is it, and how does it serve as a boon for menopausal women?

Zone 2 training refers to a specific heart rate zone, generally sitting just above the aerobic threshold and below the tempo zone. In simpler terms, it's that intensity where you work a bit harder than a comfortable jog or bike ride but can still maintain a conversation. It's a "fat-burning" zone, meaning the body primarily uses fats as its energy source.

Zone 2 and Menopausal Wonders

1. Fat Burning and Weight Management: With menopause comes a natural decline in metabolic rate and, often, an associated weight gain. Since Zone 2 training primarily targets fat metabolism, it's an excellent tool to counteract the propensity for weight gain during this life phase.

2. Cardiovascular Health: Heart health is a concern for many menopausal women due to declining estrogen levels, which protect arteries. Zone 2 training helps improve cardiovascular efficiency, promoting heart health.

3. Bone Density: Low-intensity, consistent weight-bearing activities within the Zone 2 range can aid in maintaining bone density. This is especially important for menopausal women at risk of osteoporosis.

4. Mood and Well-being: Regular Zone 2 exercise releases endorphins, those feel-good hormones that act as natural painkillers and

mood elevators. This is beneficial since many women experience mood swings and depression during menopause.

5. Stress Reduction: Menopause can be a stressful transition for many, with symptoms like hot flashes and night sweats. The consistent and rhythmic nature of Zone 2 training can have a meditative effect, reducing cortisol levels (stress hormone) and aiding in overall relaxation and stress relief.

6. Improved Sleep: Sleep disturbances are a common complaint during menopause. Zone 2 training can help regulate the body's internal clock, improving sleep quality and duration.

Understanding Metabolic Health: A Closer Look

Before we delve into the depths of Zone 2 training, let's grasp the essence of metabolic health. Traditionally, metabolic health encompassed parameters like lipid profiles, blood pressure, glucose levels, and body mass index (BMI). However, our understanding of metabolic health is evolving. It's no longer merely about ticking off boxes on a health checklist. Instead, it encompasses mitochondrial function, fitness, and longevity. We're in an era where the spotlight has shifted from metabolism being the "poor brother" in medicine to becoming a focal point in understanding and optimising health.

Metabolism, at its core, is about efficiency – the efficient conversion of potential energy in food into mechanical energy that propels our muscles and skeleton. This conversion process illuminates how our body efficiently utilises carbohydrates and fats to power our physical activities. But that's not all; it's not just about what we consume; it's also about how our bodies manage and partition fat. We'll explore the fascinating concept of the personal fat threshold and its integral role in metabolic health.

Elite Athletes as Metabolic Marvels

Why study elite athletes? It's a question that deserves a thorough answer. Elite athletes offer us a unique window into the world of metabolic health. Their bodies are finely tuned, exceptional machines designed for peak performance. In this chapter, we'll uncover why elite athletes are ideal models for understanding metabolic health. We'll delve into research demonstrating how these athletes can offer insights that apply to everyone, from weekend warriors to those embarking on their fitness journey.

From metabolic adaptations to the role of intramuscular fat, we'll unravel the science behind elite athleticism and its implications for metabolic health. It's a journey that promises to reshape our perception of what's possible for our bodies.

So, fasten your seatbelts as we embark on a journey through the intricate world of metabolic health, where exercise isn't just a lifestyle choice but a powerful tool to optimise our well-being and longevity.

Elite Athletes to Cell Powerhouses: Decoding Metabolic Mysteries

Let's start by understanding imperfection through perfection. In many ways, elite athletes represent the pinnacle of human physical performance. They are the Ferraris and Lamborghinis of the human body, finely tuned and optimised for excellence. But why study them? The answer lies in the ability to discern imperfections by knowing what perfection is. By delving into the physiology of these perfect machines, we can gain invaluable insights into understanding and addressing various diseases and interventions like exercise and nutrition.

As we explore the intricate web of metabolic health, it becomes evident that lifestyle choices play a pivotal role. Factors like sedentary lifestyles and a lack of specific cardiovascular training cannot be underestimated when it comes to the burden of cardiometabolic diseases. However, as we peer into the cellular world, mitochondria emerge as central players.

Mitochondria, often referred to as the powerhouses of cells, have taken centre stage in metabolic health. These tiny organelles convert the potential energy from carbohydrates and fats into the mechanical energy that fuels our muscles.

When we eat, about 80% of carbohydrates are metabolised in skeletal muscle, a vital organ within our bodies. This metabolic transformation predominantly occurs within the mitochondria of skeletal muscle. If these mitochondria are impaired or dysfunctional, metabolic challenges arise. Glucose, the end product of carbohydrate metabolism, must be efficiently processed. Failure to do so results in elevated blood glucose levels, a condition known as hyperglycemia. The pancreas releases insulin to combat this, which prompts glucose transport into cells.

Here's the crux – it's not just about moving glucose into cells but also about the subsequent glucose processing inside the cell. Pyruvate and glucose metabolism within the cell emerge as pivotal factors. These intricacies have immense implications, especially in the context of type 2 diabetes. While the focus has long been on hyperglycemia and insulin resistance, we must expand our understanding to encompass the entire process, including pyruvate metabolism.

Mitochondria: The Metabolic Maestro of Energy Conversion

The term 'metabolise' may sound familiar, but let's define it clearly. To metabolise means to convert substances, typically nutrients from the food we consume, into energy. This transformation process is crucial for our cells' functioning and, ultimately, our overall well-being. The central stage for this metabolic ballet is the mitochondria.

When we eat, the nutrients within our food must be metabolised into energy for our cells to utilise effectively. Glucose, for example, needs to be transformed into adenosine triphosphate (ATP), the cellular currency of energy. This intricate dance of converting nutrients to energy takes place within our mitochondria.

However, if this metabolic process falters, it poses a significant challenge to our cells. Nutrients may not be efficiently converted into energy, leading to issues like the accumulation of fats within muscle tissues. Such challenges can impact our metabolic health and our broader well-being.

Lactate's Double Life: From Metabolic Byproduct to Alzheimer's Indicator

Now, let's revisit lactate. Lactate, often misunderstood, plays a pivotal role in this metabolic orchestra. It's not just a byproduct of metabolism; it's a signalling molecule with profound implications for cellular homeostasis. When lactate accumulates excessively within a cell, it can become detrimental to its function.

Lactate's importance extends beyond metabolic health. It's become a key focus in Alzheimer's research, shedding light on the connections between diabetes, insulin resistance, mitochondrial dysfunction, and this neurodegenerative disease. Emerging research has unveiled a fascinating connection between lactate and Alzheimer's disease. While traditionally considered a waste product of metabolism, lactate is now recognised as a critical player in brain function. In Alzheimer's disease, impaired glucose metabolism in brain cells may lead to lactate buildup. This lactate can harm neuronal health, contributing to the cognitive decline observed in Alzheimer's patients. Furthermore, studies suggest that enhancing lactate utilisation by neurons through exercise and other interventions may offer a potential avenue for mitigating cognitive decline in Alzheimer's disease. This intricate link between lactate and Alzheimer's highlights the importance of understanding metabolic processes in the brain and exploring innovative strategies to combat neurodegenerative conditions.

The intricate web of metabolism, nutrients, and cellular function underscores how our choices – from exercise to nutrition – shape our metabolic health.

Mitochondria and Aging: The Vital Link to Health and Longevity

Mitochondrial dysfunction lies at the heart of many health challenges we face today. It's not just about one factor but rather the intricate interplay of various elements. As we age, our mitochondria, the tiny powerhouses within our cells, undergo several changes and challenges, such as decreased efficiency and accumulation of damage from oxidative stress. The number of mitochondria in cells may decrease as we age, which can further affect energy production. With age, the body's ability to perform autophagy efficiently may decline, accumulating malfunctioning mitochondria. The decline in mitochondrial function can reduce energy levels and increase fatigue in older individuals.

When discussing metabolic inflexibility, we refer to the body's ability to switch between burning carbohydrates and fats for energy efficiency. In a nutshell, metabolic flexibility signifies our capability to adapt to the availability of carbohydrates and fatty acids. Elite athletes and those who maintain fitness exhibit excellent metabolic flexibility. They can quickly utilise carbohydrates when they're plentiful and seamlessly switch to fatty acids when carbohydrates are scarce. This metabolic dance primarily takes place within the mitochondria.

Mitochondrial flexibility, often referred to as "metabolic flexibility," is the ability of our mitochondria to efficiently switch between using different fuels for energy production, such as carbohydrates and fats. This flexibility is crucial for maintaining metabolic health. Metabolic flexibility tends to decrease with age. Our mitochondria may become less adept at switching between fuel sources as we age. This reduced flexibility can make it more challenging for the body to adapt to changes in diet or energy demands.

One aspect of metabolic flexibility involves the ability to burn fats for energy. This decline can impact overall metabolic health and contribute to age-related metabolic disorders. With age, there is often a decreased capacity to utilise fats as a fuel source, which can contribute to metabolic issues and obesity. Aging can lead to a greater reliance on glucose as the primary energy source, even when fats are available. This shift towards glucose metabolism can be associated with insulin resistance and an increased risk of metabolic diseases like type 2 diabetes. This poses a metabolic challenge, leading to elevated blood glucose levels and fat deposition in muscles and adipose tissue.

Let's connect the dots to conditions like fatty liver disease, type 2 diabetes, and cardiovascular disease. These diseases are often multifactorial, with various elements working together. Nevertheless, mitochondrial decay or dysfunction is frequently at the root of the problem. Mitochondrial dysfunction disrupts the efficient metabolism of nutrients, setting the stage for disease. It can result in hyperglycemia (elevated blood glucose levels) and increased fat storage in muscles and adipose tissue. However, pinpointing the precise cause of mitochondrial dysfunction is complex.

One thing is clear: physical activity is pivotal in maintaining mitochondrial function. Exercise is both the cause of mitochondrial decay when absent and the solution to improve mitochondrial function when present. Unfortunately, most of the older population leads sedentary lives, contributing to widespread mitochondrial dysfunction.

Comprehending Energy Zones

Understanding how exercise intensity impacts energy utilisation and production is crucial for optimising performance and health. Let's delve into the various energy zones or exercise intensities and how they relate to the substrates used for energy production:

1. Zone 1 (Low Intensity): In this zone, characterised by light activities like an easy walk or a gentle bike ride, the body predominantly relies on fat as its primary energy source. However, it's important to note that glucose is still used to some extent, dispelling the misconception that glucose utilisation is absent at low intensities.

2. Zone 2 (Moderate Intensity): As exercise intensity increases to a moderate level, glucose utilisation increases as exercise intensity rises, but fat is still used as a significant energy source. This is because glucose can be converted into energy more quickly, making it a valuable resource for sustained effort.

3. Zone 3 (Threshold Intensity): You're exercising at a level just below your lactate threshold in this zone. The lactate threshold represents the point at which lactate production in muscles increases significantly. The body relies heavily on carbohydrates, primarily glucose, as

the primary energy source at this intensity. Fat utilisation is still present but less than in Zone 1 or 2.

4. Zone 4 (High Intensity): Zone 4 corresponds to high-intensity efforts where the body's demand for immediate energy is paramount. Glucose becomes the predominant source of fuel, and fat utilisation decreases significantly. This zone is often associated with intense interval training or near-maximal efforts.

5. Zone 5 (Maximum Intensity): At the highest exercise intensity levels, the body relies almost exclusively on glucose to meet the energy demands. This is typically seen in short, all-out efforts or sprinting. Fat utilisation is minimal in Zone 5.

6. Zone 6 (Anaerobic): In Zone 6, exercise intensity reaches a point where the body's demand for ATP production surpasses what can be provided by aerobic metabolism. The muscles tap into their stored ATP reserves and involve pure anaerobic metabolism, where the body taps into stored ATP and the phosphocreatine system for energy. This zone is associated with sprinting or very high-intensity efforts lasting a few minutes.

Regarding the production of ATP from glucose and fat, while more ATP can be derived from fat per mole oxidised, the critical difference lies in the rate of ATP production. Glucose allows for faster ATP production compared to fat. This speed in ATP production becomes crucial as exercise intensity increases because the muscles require energy more rapidly.

It's important to note that the transition between these zones is not abrupt but relatively gradual. The body dynamically adjusts its fuel selection based on exercise intensity and duration. The key takeaway is that different exercise intensities elicit distinct metabolic responses and influence the substrates used for energy production. Understanding these zones can help tailor training strategies for specific fitness goals and optimise performance.

Fueling Fitness: The Science of Exercise Intensity Zones

These exercise intensity zones are not rigidly defined but represent a continuum, with the body dynamically adjusting its fuel sources based on the intensity and duration of exercise. Understanding these zones can guide training strategies to achieve specific fitness goals and optimise performance.

At lower intensities, the body primarily relies on the oxidative phosphorylation system, an aerobic energy production system within the mitochondria. Regarding the production of ATP from glucose and fat, while more ATP can be derived from fat per mole oxidised, the critical difference lies in the rate of ATP production. Glucose allows for faster ATP production compared to fat. This speed in ATP production becomes crucial as exercise intensity increases because the muscles require energy more rapidly.

The preference for fat at lower intensities can be attributed to our evolutionary history. Fat provides a more extensive and long-lasting energy reserve, which is essential for endurance activities and survival. In contrast, glycogen (stored glucose) is relatively limited in storage capacity, making it a valuable resource that the body tries to conserve.

The significance of Zone 2 is because it is the point of Maximum Fat Oxidation. Exercising in this zone provides a specific and direct stimulus to the mitochondria, leading to adaptations and improvements in mitochondrial function and efficiency. This can have a positive impact on overall endurance and aerobic capacity.

Elite Edge: Lactate Mastery in High-Performance Athletes

Elite athletes often produce more lactate because their glycolytic system, known as the "turbo," is highly efficient. This efficiency allows them to use more glucose for energy production, increasing lactate production during high-intensity exercise.

However, the critical difference is that these elite athletes possess robust mitochondrial function and effective lactate clearance mechanisms. Elite athletes can oxidise more significant amounts of glucose during high-intensity exercise, producing higher lactate. This glycolytic efficiency is beneficial for quick bursts of energy needed in various sports. What sets elite athletes apart is their ability to rapidly clear lactate. They can transport lactate from fast-twitch muscle fibres, primarily produced during intense efforts, to adjacent slow-twitch muscle fibres. These slow-twitch fibres, with their well-functioning mitochondria, effectively oxidise the lactate.

To facilitate lactate clearance, transporters play a crucial role. Elite athletes often have more efficient lactate transporters that shuttle lactate away from the muscles where it's produced to areas where it can be effectively used or cleared. So, it's not that elite athletes produce less lactate; they may produce more due to their superior glycolytic capacity. However, their ability to clear and utilise lactate efficiently sets them apart and allows them to perform at high levels during intense exercise.

This combination of glycolytic prowess and efficient lactate management contributes to the exceptional performance of elite athletes, particularly in sports that demand bursts of high-intensity effort.

Energy Dance: Mastering Lactate Clearance for Peak Performance

In the world of exercise physiology, the concept of lactate clearance holds a pivotal role in understanding how our bodies respond to different forms of training. To break it down, two main types of transporters are involved: MCT4 and MCT1. MCT4, often called the "doors," is crucial in shuttling lactate out of fast-twitch muscle fibres. These fibres are predominantly engaged during high-intensity activities like sprinting or resistance training.

To optimise lactate clearance, it's essential to stimulate these fast-twitch muscle fibres through intense training. This enhances glycolytic capacity, essentially your body's turbo mode, and improves the efficiency of MCT4 transporters, allowing them to remove lactate from the muscle cells more effectively.

On the other hand, we have the slow-twitch muscle fibres, which are the primary focus during lower-intensity workouts, often categorised as "zone two" training. These fibres are highly efficient at burning fat and are rich in mitochondria, our cellular powerhouses. Interestingly, MCT1 transporters are also present in these slow-twitch fibres.

So, what's the significance of stimulating these slow-twitch fibres during your training routine? Well, it's twofold. First, it enhances mitochondrial function, a critical factor in overall health and longevity. Second, it contributes to lactate clearance. By engaging these fibres, you create a dynamic Push-Pull system where lactate is shuttled out of fast-twitch fibres and into slow-twitch ones. This process helps keep lactate levels in check and utilises lactate as an energy source, further optimising your workouts.

This intricate dance of lactate clearance and mitochondrial function might sound complex, but it's essential to grasp when designing your exercise regimen. Whether you're an elite athlete aiming for peak performance or pursuing better metabolic health, understanding how different training intensities impact these processes is vital. It's about identifying your strengths and weaknesses and tailoring your workouts accordingly.

In the ever-evolving world of sports science, this paradigm of lactate clearance and mitochondrial optimisation has proven its worth. It's a concept that's brought success to elite athletes and improved the lives of individuals with chronic health conditions. As we continue to explore the boundaries of exercise physiology, remember that the path to better performance and longevity often begins by asking, "Which energy system do you want to stimulate today?"

Unlocking the Secret of Ageless Energy: Why VO2 Max is Only Half the Story!

In the quest for optimal health and fitness, we often fixate on metrics like VO2 max, the gold standard for measuring cardiorespiratory fitness. While VO2 max is undoubtedly a valuable tool, our journey into the world of cellular biology reveals that there's more to the story.

Consider the intriguing case of two athletes both reaching 350 Watts during their exercise routines. One displays eight millimoles of lactate, while the other registers just three or four millimoles. Surprisingly, despite having similar VO2 max values, their lactate levels differ significantly. This revelation prompts us to dive deeper into the cellular level, where the real magic happens. Here, we uncover a fascinating truth—VO2 max, though crucial, merely scratches the surface of our understanding of health and fitness.

In the last two decades, researchers have focused on the microscopic world of cellular biology, unearthing hidden treasures that hold the key to our well-being. Central to this exploration is the enigmatic mitochondrion, often called the powerhouse of our cells. Mitochondria, the queens of cellular life, deserve our attention. They orchestrate a symphony of metabolic processes, ensuring our bodies have the energy to thrive. But when it comes to stimulating these mitochondrial powerhouses through Zone 2 training, what are we aiming for?

The answer lies in a delicate balance—improving both the function and number of mitochondria within our muscle fibres. While the debate between function and quantity persists, evidence suggests that function takes precedence. A well-functioning mitochondria can be a game-changer; this is where our journey begins. Studies have shown that individuals with type 2 diabetes or obesity often have lower muscle mitochondrial content. The sedentary lifestyle that has become the norm in modern society exacerbates this decline. The good news is that exercise can work wonders, even at the cellular level. Research by esteemed scientists has demonstrated that aerobic training can triple the number of mitochondria within muscle tissue. This transformation includes an increase in quantity and an improvement in size and function. These findings underscore the remarkable plasticity of our skeletal muscles.

Unlock Your Inner Mitochondrial Superhero: Transform Your Health with Ancient Wisdom!

We must recognise that we are not bound by a fixed number of mitochondria from birth. Instead, we possess the power to influence their fate. If years of sedentary living have depleted our mitochondrial army, we can embark on a journey to rebuild it through exercise.

Understanding that our genes have not evolved to thrive in a sedentary environment is crucial. On the contrary, we are genetically predisposed to be physically active. The rise of sedentary lifestyles, driven by technological progress, has led to a surge in non-communicable diseases.

To put this into perspective, let's examine the lifestyles of primitive civilisations that still exist in our world today. The Hadza hunter-gatherers in Tanzania and the Tsimane people in Bolivia offer us a glimpse into a life untouched by modern sedentary habits. These populations have maintained their traditional lifestyles, offering a unique perspective on health and fitness. Remarkably, the Hadza and Tsimane populations exhibit obesity rates as low as two per cent and have only one per cent prevalence of type 2 diabetes. Their cardiovascular health is exceptional, with the lowest observed levels of atherosclerosis plaque among any human population. These findings underscore the importance of a well-functioning mitochondrial system in energy production.

Our exploration of cellular biology and mitochondrial health unravels a complex and captivating narrative. While VO2 max remains a valuable metric, our understanding of health and fitness has evolved to encompass the cellular intricacies that dictate our well-being. Mitochondria, the unsung heroes within our cells, hold the key to our vitality. Through exercise and proper care, we can rekindle the power of our mitochondria and embark on a journey to optimal health.

Zone 2 Training Secrets: Transform Your Body and Boost Metabolism!

Zone 2, in essence, is the exercise intensity where one can maximise the improvement of mitochondrial function. It's not the only beneficial zone, but it has proven particularly effective in enhancing mitochondrial function, which is essential for optimal metabolic health. The critical question arises: How can you identify and implement Zone 2 training into your fitness routine? The good news is that it's not as complicated as it may sound.

Identifying Zone 2

You can use various methods to determine your Zone 2, including heart rate monitoring, power metres on bikes, or simply gauging your perceived exertion. Heart rate monitoring is widespread, and Zone 2 typically corresponds to about 60-70% of your maximum heart rate. It's an intensity where you can still maintain a conversation comfortably. You should feel challenged but not push yourself to the limit.

Zone 2 Training Frequency

So, how often should you engage in Zone 2 training to promote mitochondrial health and metabolic fitness? Ideally, incorporating Zone 2 workouts into your routine three to four times a week can yield significant benefits. This doesn't mean every session has to be a gruelling workout; even moderately paced activities count.

Duration of Zone 2 Workouts

The duration of your Zone 2 workouts can vary based on your fitness level. Beginners might start with 30-45 minutes per session, gradually increasing the duration as their fitness improves. More experienced individuals can aim for 60-90 minutes or even longer for endurance.

Integrating Zone 2 into Your Routine

Incorporating Zone 2 workouts into your fitness regimen doesn't require a significant overhaul. Consider activities like brisk walking, cycling, swimming, or even hiking. Maintaining that sustainable, conversational pace while staying consistent with your training frequency is key.

Customising Zone 2 Training

Keep in mind that everyone's fitness level and goals are different. You can customise your Zone 2 training to align with your specific objectives. Whether you're training for a marathon, looking to lose weight, or simply aiming to boost overall health, Zone 2 can be tailored to suit your needs.

Monitoring Progress

Lastly, monitoring your progress as you embark on your Zone 2 journey is essential. Track your workouts, heart rate, and how you feel during and after each session. Over time, you should notice improvements in your endurance, fat-burning capacity, and overall well-being.

Choosing Your Zone 2 Weapon

Now that you know where to find Zone 2, it's time to choose your weapon of choice. The good news is there's no one-size-fits-all approach. Whether you prefer jogging through serene parks, cycling along scenic routes, or swimming in tranquil waters, you can adapt these activities to fit your Zone 2 training regimen. We aim to keep your heart rate within the Zone 2 range, regardless of your selected activity.

Building Your Zone 2 Routine

Building a Zone 2 training routine requires consistency and patience. You might wonder how much time you must dedicate to reap the benefits. While the guidelines suggest a minimum of 150 minutes per week, viewing this as a starting point rather than a final destination is essential. Recent research suggests that more extended periods say 300 to 400 minutes a week, could provide superior results.

However, the real key is the total time spent and the quality of your Zone 2 sessions. We recommend striving for continuous workouts within your Zone 2 range. This means staying in that aerobic sweet spot for a significant portion of your session. Whether you can achieve this in one more extended session or several shorter ones throughout the week depends on your schedule and preferences.

Maximising the Benefits

By committing to Zone 2 training, you can unlock many health advantages. Notably, it promotes mitochondrial biogenesis, essentially increasing the number and efficiency of your mitochondria. This leads to better energy production, improved fat oxidation, and enhanced metabolic health. Furthermore, Zone 2 training aids in fat loss, encouraging your body to use stored fat as a primary fuel source. This can be particularly beneficial for those aiming to shed excess weight or improve body composition.

Zone 2 training isn't just about improving your athletic performance; it's about transforming your metabolic health and enhancing longevity. We've seen remarkable transformations in individuals who've embraced this training approach, even in their later years. It's never too late to start and experience the positive changes it can bring to your life.

Timing Your Zone 2 Sessions

While the concept of Zone 2 training itself is transformative, the timing of these sessions can make a significant difference. The question that often arises is, "When should I schedule my Zone 2 workouts for maximum benefit?" The answer, of course, varies from person to person due to individual schedules and preferences. However, let's explore a few key considerations.

Morning Glory: Many individuals find that engaging in Zone 2 training in the morning provides a refreshing start to their day. It can boost alertness, increase metabolic rate, and set a positive tone for the hours ahead. This is especially beneficial if you're targeting fat-burning as a primary goal.

Lunchtime Lift: Some prefer the midday slot for their Zone 2 sessions. A lunchtime workout can serve as an excellent break from the workday, helping to rejuvenate both body and mind. However, managing your time effectively is crucial to ensure you can complete the session without rushing.

Evening Ease: Evening Zone 2 training can be a fantastic way to unwind after a day of responsibilities. It's also an ideal option for those who may not be morning people. However, remember that exercising too close to bedtime may affect your sleep quality, so it's best to leave some buffer time.

Individual Variations

The best timing for your Zone 2 sessions depends on your body's natural rhythms, lifestyle, and preferences. It's essential to listen to your body and find a routine that you can sustain over the long term. Consistency remains the key, and if you're more likely to stick to your sessions at a particular time, that's likely the best time for you.

Daylight and Environment

Consider your surroundings when choosing your Zone 2 training time. Some may prefer outdoor sessions during daylight hours to soak in vitamin D and enjoy natural scenery. Others might opt for indoor workouts, allowing for more controlled conditions. Both options have their merits, and it's up to you to determine which aligns best with your goals and lifestyle.

Combining with Other Activities

One fascinating aspect of Zone 2 training is its adaptability to various activities. You can incorporate it into your daily routine by choosing active commuting, like cycling or brisk walking to work. This not only saves time but also integrates fitness seamlessly into your life. Remember that your Zone 2 training doesn't need to be a rigid, separate entity in your schedule. It can blend with other activities, making it even more sustainable in the long run.

In summary, Zone 2 training is a powerful tool to enhance mitochondrial function, boost metabolic health, and achieve fitness goals. It's a sustainable, practical approach that can benefit individuals of all fitness levels. As you embark on your Zone 2 journey, remember that consistency and patience are key to reaping the rewards of improved mitochondrial health and overall well-being.

The Fasted State Dilemma

One question that often arises is whether performing Zone 2 training in a fasted state or following a high-fat, low-carb diet can enhance fat oxidation and, in turn, boost mitochondrial adaptations. While these strategies hold promise, they come with important caveats. Fasting and exercising in tandem can be a double-edged sword. On the one hand, it may stimulate fat oxidation due to reduced glycogen availability. However, caution must be exercised to prevent overexertion and potential catabolism. Managing exercise intensity and frequency is crucial in this scenario.

Moreover, the idea of restricting carbohydrates to promote fat oxidation is not without its complexities. The shift in substrate utilisation observed during fasting or low-carb diets may be more of a metabolic artefact related to glycogen depletion. Thus, the long-term efficacy of these approaches in improving mitochondrial function is still under scrutiny.

The Mitochondrial Puzzle

The key to enhancing fat oxidation and mitochondrial function lies in improving your mitochondria's efficiency. While dietary strategies may play a role, exercise remains the primary driver of these adaptations. Focusing on regular, consistent Zone 2 training is the most reliable path to success.

Supplements and Their Controversy

Recently, supplements like urolithin A have garnered attention for their purported ability to boost mitochondrial function. Urolithin A is a compound naturally produced by our gut bacteria from certain polyphenols found in berries and pomegranates. However, the claims surrounding such supplements should be met with cautious scrutiny. The scientific consensus regarding their efficacy remains limited; anecdotal reports often precede robust evidence. Additionally, individual responses to supplements can vary widely, making it challenging to generalise their impact.

Other supplements, such as nicotinamide mononucleotide (NMN), which is a precursor of NAD (nicotinamide adenine dinucleotide), have been marketed for their potential to enhance cellular function. Nevertheless, the effects of such supplements are still a subject of ongoing research, and their long-term implications are yet to be fully understood.

The Placebo Factor

It's important to note that the placebo effect can significantly influence perceived benefits from supplements. Many individuals report remarkable improvements shortly after starting a new supplement regimen, only for the effects to diminish over time. This phenomenon underscores the need for rigorous scientific scrutiny and long-term studies to establish the true efficacy of supplements. As we delve deeper into the realm of nutrition and supplementation, remember that exercise remains the cornerstone of mitochondrial health. While these adjuncts may hold promise, they should complement, not replace, your commitment to Zone 2 training. A balanced and evidence-based approach is key in the quest for optimal health and fitness.

Striking a Balance: The Zone 3 and Zone 4 Conundrum

Let's navigate the intricate terrain of exercise intensity beyond Zone 2. While Zone 2 has taken centre stage in our discussions, it's essential to recognise that cardiovascular training is not confined to a single zone. Let's explore the nuances and significance of Zone 3 and Zone 4 in your quest for optimal health and fitness.

Throughout our journey, we've emphasised the pivotal role of Zone 2 training in fostering mitochondrial health and enhancing metabolic function. However, it's crucial to acknowledge that the exercise landscape is far from one-dimensional. A healthy and balanced training regimen comprises various intensities and modalities.

Zone 3 and Zone 4 are often labelled as "no man's land" or dismissed as "junk volume." This oversimplification fails to capture their significance in the broader context of cardiovascular training. These higher-intensity zones have their unique roles and benefits.

Zone 3 serves as a bridge between the aerobic and anaerobic realms. While it may lack the mitochondrial focus of Zone 2, it plays a crucial role in improving lactate threshold and aerobic power. Embracing Zone 3 workouts periodically can help you push your boundaries and achieve greater fitness gains.

Zone 4 represents the threshold of high-intensity training. While it strays from the comfortable, conversational pace of Zone 2, it offers substantial benefits in terms of anaerobic capacity, explosive power, and overall cardiovascular fitness. Although not a zone to reside in exclusively, strategically incorporating Zone 4 sessions can enhance your performance.

The Comprehensive Cardiovascular Approach

To optimise your cardiovascular fitness, embracing a well-rounded training approach is essential. Zone 2 remains the foundation, nurturing your mitochondrial health and metabolic efficiency. However, Zone 3 and Zone 4 sessions add depth and diversity to your training, allowing you to target different aspects of fitness.

Balancing Act

In the pursuit of fitness excellence, balance is critical. Don't confine yourself to a single zone, and avoid extremes. Instead, craft a training plan that integrates Zone 2 as the cornerstone while strategically sprinkling in Zone 3 and Zone 4. This balanced approach can unlock your full potential and keep your workouts engaging. For women embarking on the journey through shifting hormonal landscapes, when time is a precious resource, I suggest emphasising Zone 2 training while incorporating a resistance training regimen. This combination can lay the foundation for a robust Zone 2 base. Conversely, in situations where time is more abundant, delving into other training zones can propel one towards attaining a remarkably superior and elite physique.

As we navigate the intricacies of cardiovascular training, remember that your journey is unique. Your training should align with your goals, preferences, and physical condition. The world of exercise is multifaceted, offering various tools to sculpt your ideal fitness regimen.

Chapter 14
The Swinging Pendulum of Hormone Replacement Therapy

For many years, Hormone Replacement Therapy (HRT) was hailed as the go-to treatment for menopausal symptoms, offering women relief from hot flashes, night sweats, and other disruptive experiences. The pendulum swung decisively in favour of HRT in the 80s and 90s, with doctors readily prescribing it as a panacea for menopause-related woes. However, the landmark Women's Health Initiative (WHI) study dramatically altered this perspective.

The Women's Health Initiative (WHI) Hormone Therapy Trials began in 1991 and originally planned to run until 2005. However, the oestrogen-plus-progestin arm of the study was halted in July 2002, and the oestrogen-alone arm was halted in February 2004. Both parts were stopped early because it was determined that the risks outweighed the benefits. Follow-up studies have continued to assess the long-term health outcomes of the participants. Therefore, while the main trials were conducted over approximately 11 to 13 years, follow-up analyses are ongoing.

The study's findings on the potential risks of HRT, including an increased likelihood of heart attacks, strokes, and certain types of cancer, sent shockwaves through the medical community and led many healthcare providers to become cautious or even sceptical of HRT.

As a result, the pendulum swung sharply in the opposite direction, with HRT becoming somewhat of a medical pariah. Women were suddenly caught in a quandary, torn between enduring menopausal symptoms and taking on potential health risks. The journey to decide upon HRT is mired in ambiguity, with experts presenting compelling arguments from opposing viewpoints.

Today, the pendulum seems to be settling somewhere in the middle. A nuanced understanding of HRT is emerging, fueled by further studies and real-world experiences. It's becoming increasingly clear that the suitability of HRT depends on various factors, including a woman's specific symptoms, overall health, and lifestyle choices. As new formulations and methods of administration become available, like transdermal patch estradiol and micronized progesterone, both clinicians and patients have more options to consider.

Therefore, it is essential for women to be informed and proactive, working closely with healthcare providers who are experts in menopause management. An individualised approach, focused on personal symptoms and risks, is the current mantra in optimising menopause treatment.

The Women's Health Initiative (WHI)

Diving into the groundbreaking research that reshaped perceptions on Hormone Replacement Therapy: The Women's Health Initiative (WHI) remains the most comprehensive study ever conducted on post-menopausal women. Initiated in 1981, this expansive study involved over 160,000 women across the United States, ranging in age from 50 to 79. Its primary aims were:

1. Assessing the benefits and risks of menopausal hormone therapy.

2. Investigating the effects of calcium and vitamin D supplementation.

3. Evaluating if a low-fat diet could lower the risks of breast and colorectal cancer.

In addition, over half of the participants were part of an observational cohort designed to study other risk factors and preventive measures against chronic diseases in post-menopausal women.

Decoding WHI: Hormone Therapy Trials and Their Implications

The hormone therapy trials within the WHI were particularly intriguing. These were divided into two categories: one for women with an intact uterus, incorporating both oestrogen and progestin; and another for women who had undergone hysterectomy, utilising oestrogen alone. The trials aimed to clarify the balance of benefits and risks of hormone therapy when used for preventing chronic diseases like heart attacks and strokes. The study was not focused on evaluating the efficacy of hormone therapy for treating symptoms like hot flashes and night sweats, as this had already been established.

WHI Insights: Calcium, Vitamin D, and Fracture Prevention

Another focal point of the WHI was to examine whether calcium and vitamin D supplementation could effectively reduce fractures. While previous trials had primarily involved women with osteoporosis or low bone mineral density, the WHI looked at a broader range of bone mineral densities to evaluate the potential benefits of calcium and vitamin D in fracture prevention.

WHI Decoded: Low-Fat Diets vs. Cancer Risks

The low-fat dietary modification trial within the WHI aimed to resolve the long-debated issue of whether a low-fat diet could lower the risks of breast and colorectal cancer. This was done through a randomised clinical trial and is a key contribution to understanding women's nutritional needs and risks related to chronic diseases.

Here's a summary of its findings based on a low-fat diet:

1. Heart Disease: The WHI found that a low-fat diet did not significantly reduce the risk of coronary heart disease, stroke, or cardiovascular disease in postmenopausal women.

2. Breast Cancer: The study found no statistically significant reduction in breast cancer risk for women who were advised to follow a low-fat diet.

3. Colorectal Cancer: No significant difference in the risk of colorectal cancer was observed between women on a low-fat diet and those on a standard diet.

4. Weight: Women on the low-fat diet lost weight in the first year but regained some weight in the following years. Overall, the difference in weight between the two groups was modest.

5. Other Health Outcomes: No significant differences were noted in the risk for other cancers, type 2 diabetes, or fractures between the two groups.

In conclusion, the WHI dietary modification trial found that a low-fat diet did not substantially affect the risk of heart disease, most cancers, or other major chronic diseases among postmenopausal women. So it perplexes me why some doctors advocate a low-fat diet for women approaching menopause when their benefits have long been questioned decades ago.

WHI Unraveled: The Double-Edged Sword of Hormone Therapy

The Women's Health Initiative (WHI) study significantly altered perceptions and practices surrounding hormone therapy. Before the WHI, observational studies led many to believe that hormone therapy would lower risks of heart attacks and all-cause mortality and even improve cognitive function. However, the WHI results revealed that, particularly for oestrogen plus progestin therapy, the risks seemed to outweigh the benefits in preventing chronic diseases.

On the risk side, there was a significant increase in strokes, pulmonary embolisms, a borderline increase in heart attacks, and a notable rise in breast cancer cases. It's crucial to note that these adverse events were predominantly observed in women in their late 60s and 70s, emphasising the role of age in these outcomes. On the benefit side, the study showed more than a 30% reduction in hip fractures and a decrease in colorectal cancer, specifically with oestrogen plus progestin.

These results led to a dramatic drop in hormone therapy prescriptions by over 70%. While this may have curbed inappropriate use, it also halted some appropriate use, particularly among younger women going through menopause who were experiencing distressing symptoms like hot flashes and night sweats. These women could have had a more favourable benefit-risk ratio, compared to older women in the WHI.

Age Bias and Other Flaws: Delving into the WHI's Oestrogen-Only Therapy Study Outcomes

Regarding flaws in the WHI study, one commonly cited issue is the age of the participants. The average age was around 61 to 63, which likely skewed results, particularly since younger women going through menopause might have different risk profiles.

Regarding oestrogen-only therapy in women with hysterectomies, the outcomes seemed more balanced. While there was about a 40% increase in stroke, most other outcomes were neutral between the estrogen-only and placebo arms. Also, this therapy led to approximately a one-third reduction in hip fractures.

Evolution of Hormone Therapy: From WHI Concerns to Modern Formulations

Fast forward 20 years, and we have new formulations like bioidentical hormones, oral oestrogen, and micronised progesterone. Existing research, both observational and smaller randomised trials, suggests that transdermal oestrogen might offer a more favourable benefit-risk profile, particularly in reducing thrombotic risks, such as blood clots in the legs and lungs, compared to oral oestrogen. However, it's less clear if the risk of stroke could be entirely avoided, but it's plausible that it could be reduced.

The WHI did touch on ovarian cancer, but the numbers were too small for a definitive conclusion. However, there was a borderline increase in risk associated with both forms of hormone therapy. The types of progestins used in the study are different from those in birth control pills and IUDs, which also have clotting risks but at higher doses. The risk of clotting is particularly elevated with oral formulations that affect the liver's synthesis of clotting factors.

Today, newer formulations like transdermal estradiol and micronised progesterone are preferred, but oral hormone therapy is still in use. It's important to remember that sometimes randomised clinical trials can yield surprising results, and we don't have large-scale trials for the newer formulations like transdermal estradiol and micronised progesterone.

Minding the Gap: Rethinking Menopause Education in Medicine

As an aesthetics and anti-ageing doctor with an interest in menopause, I will be the first to admit that the mainstream medical curriculum has significant gaps in this area. From medical school to internships, residencies, and fellowships, the education on menopause and hormone therapy is insufficient.

Many clinicians emerge from their training with an inadequate understanding of how to discuss the risks, benefits, and alternatives of hormone therapy with patients. This lack of information makes engaging in shared decision-making, properly evaluating symptoms, and making clinically appropriate decisions challenging.

The neglect of menopause management in medical training is concerning, given that it affects a large patient population segment. Women live 40% or more of their lives in the postmenopausal phase, facing increased risks of chronic diseases such as bone loss, osteoporosis, heart disease, Type 2 diabetes, stroke, and various cancers. Despite these critical issues, menopause management, which includes treating symptoms like hot flashes and lifestyle interventions for disease prevention, receives scant attention.

Regarding health promotion, regular physical activity stands out as a potent preventive measure against a host of conditions, including heart disease, stroke, osteoporosis, Type 2 diabetes, and several forms of cancer. Despite its numerous benefits for emotional well-being and sleep quality, most patients don't receive adequate counselling on physical activity.

The current healthcare system is more of a 'disease care system,' with little emphasis on preventive measures like diet, physical activity, and smoking cessation. Even though the adage 'prevention is better than cure' is widely recognised, it doesn't receive the attention it deserves in healthcare settings, particularly concerning chronic disease prevention.

In the context of the Nurses' Health Study, we've had the opportunity to examine how lifestyle and behavioural choices are closely tied to the risk of various chronic diseases, including heart attacks, strokes, Type 2 diabetes, and multiple forms of cancer. The Nurses' Health Study (NHS) is a series of extensive studies initiated in 1976, examining the long-term effects of nutrition, hormones, and other factors on health and disease in nurses. Led by investigators at institutions like Harvard Medical School and Brigham and Women's Hospital, the study started with 121,700 female registered nurses aged between 30 and 55 from 11 U.S. states. Initial focus areas included contraception use, smoking, cancer, and cardiovascular disease, with surveys distributed biennially. In 1980, the study integrated a dietary questionnaire, recognising diet's role in chronic disease. Over the years, they began collecting physical samples and verifying morbidity using various methods.

Unraveling Health Secrets from the Nurses' Health Study

The Nurses' Health Study II, initiated in 1989, zeroed in on women's health and the long-term effects of oral contraceptives, expanding later to broader health metrics. By 1999, 30,000 nurses had provided samples, focusing on hormone levels and their influence on disease risk. This study even led to a second-generation follow-up named the Growing Up Today Study.

The third iteration, Nurses' Health Study 3, launched in 2010, widened its participant base to include both men and women and expanded its geographic reach to Canada. Driven by a diverse team of researchers, the study continues to be a cornerstone in understanding health and chronic diseases.

The studies identified various correlations, or statistical links, between environmental factors and potential health risks.

1. Smoking: Found to increase the risk of cardiovascular disease (CVD), colorectal and pancreatic cancer, psoriasis, multiple sclerosis, type 2 diabetes, and eye diseases.

2. Trans Fats: Consumption was linked to an increased risk of CVD. This connection led to the inclusion of trans fats on U.S. food labels in 2003 and the FDA's decision to label partially hydrogenated oils as unsafe.

3. Obesity: Positively linked to a higher risk of CVD, breast and pancreatic cancer, psoriasis, multiple sclerosis, gallstones, type 2 diabetes, and eye diseases.

4. Postmenopausal Hormone Therapy: Found to reduce the risk of CVD. However, using combination hormones (progesterone and estrogen) showed an increased risk of breast cancer.

5. Oral Contraceptives: Demonstrated a reduced risk of ovarian cancer. The study found no significant link between oral contraceptives and breast cancer risk, and neither current nor past use showed a strong correlation with CVD.

6. Exercise: Showed a link to improved breast cancer survival rates. Physical activity was associated with a reduced risk of CVD and type 2 diabetes.

The study also delved into various other factors, such as diet, coffee intake, and sleep patterns, producing a wide range of findings.

Unfortunately, these vital aspects of health—diet, physical activity, and overall lifestyle—are often overlooked. Before pursuing medical treatments, one should first consider non-medical interventions like diet and exercise, as well as minimising lifestyle behaviours that could increase disease risk.

Hormone Therapy in Women's Health: Weighing the Benefits and Risks

So, let's delve into hormone therapy, especially its role in women's health. Before the results of the Women's Health Initiative, hormone therapy was almost universally recommended for preventing heart attacks, strokes, and cognitive decline. Even women without menopausal symptoms were advised to undergo hormone therapy as they aged. However, the pendulum swung in the opposite direction after the 2002 findings of the oestrogen plus progestin trial, with many considering hormone therapy as having an unfavourable benefit-to-risk ratio.

Now, the consensus is becoming more nuanced. Hormone therapy may be beneficial for some women but not all. It is particularly relevant for those experiencing severe menopausal symptoms that affect their quality of life. Importantly, it should be considered on a case-by-case basis, taking into account factors such as the individual's age, health status, the severity of symptoms, and potential contraindications like a history of blood clots, breast cancer, or high cardiovascular risk.

So, should women take hormones for prevention against conditions like dementia, bone issues, or cardiovascular diseases? The current medical stance suggests that hormone therapy is most appropriate for women in early menopause suffering from moderate to severe menopausal symptoms, particularly when these symptoms disturb their sleep, and who do not have contraindications like a high risk of cardiovascular disease or breast cancer.

Thus, the decision to undergo hormone therapy should be personalised, made in consultation with a healthcare provider, and based on a comprehensive understanding of the benefits and risks involved.

The use of hormone therapy to prevent heart disease, stroke, cognitive decline, or osteoporotic fractures remains a contentious issue. It's generally not advised for disease prevention. Some clinicians may consider hormone therapy for osteoporosis prevention in women at higher risk and with no contraindications. The prevailing view is that hormone therapy is most appropriate for managing moderate to severe menopausal symptoms like hot flashes and night sweats rather than for disease prevention in asymptomatic women.

Alternative treatments exist for other health issues like osteoporotic fractures and heart disease. These include statins for cardiovascular risk management and lifestyle changes such as maintaining a healthy diet and regular physical exercise. Furthermore, hormone therapy has not proven beneficial for women in age groups where these health conditions are most prevalent, namely women in their 60s, 70s, and 80s.

In terms of defining "early menopause," according to the Women's Health Initiative findings, the benefit-risk profile for hormone therapy is more favourable for women in their 50s or within ten years of menopausal onset. Most randomised trials on hormone therapy have been conducted on postmenopausal women, meaning they've had their last menstrual cycle and gone a year or more without menstruating. The utility of hormone therapy during the perimenopausal phase has not been rigorously studied in randomised trials.

Bioidentical Hormone Therapy: Making Informed Choices in Menopause Management

When it comes to hormone therapy, particularly for menopausal symptoms, it's essential to distinguish between FDA-approved formulations like transdermal patch estradiol and micronised progesterone, and compounded versions. The FDA-approved options have undergone rigorous testing for purity, consistent content, and absence of contaminants.

Many women may assume that "bioidentical" automatically means they should seek a compounding pharmacy, but FDA-approved bioidentical options like transdermal patch estradiol are available. These are especially relevant for women in early menopause within the first ten years following their last menstrual cycle. The focus should be on both quality-of-life issues, like symptom management, and hard clinical outcomes, such as rates of heart attacks and strokes, as well as cognitive function.

Conducting trials on these newer formulations will require substantial investment, and the results might not even be relevant by the time they are concluded, given how quickly medical treatments can evolve. For example, the Women's Health Initiative had trials with 27,000 participants, and a new study would require even more participants due to fewer clinical events in early menopause.

If you're a woman considering hormone therapy, it's crucial to consult a clinician with expertise in menopause management. Treatment options should be discussed thoroughly, including hormonal and non-hormonal therapies.

It's imperative to seek treatment if you're experiencing moderate to severe symptoms that impact your quality of life. While hormone therapy appears to be the most effective, other viable treatments exist. If you have a strong family history of osteoporosis, this should also be part of your discussion with your healthcare provider. However, hormone therapy should not be initiated solely to prevent heart attacks, strokes, or cognitive decline if you're not experiencing menopausal symptoms.

Finally, aside from medical treatments, lifestyle and nutritional supplements can also help manage menopausal symptoms, as long as they are backed by scientific evidence. There are multiple treatment approaches, and women must find a healthcare provider to guide them through these complex decisions.

Chapter 15
Navigating Menopause with Nature's Aid

M enopause is a unique journey for every woman. Choosing the right supplements to alleviate specific symptoms can be a personal exploration. In this chapter, we'll delve into four critical concerns during menopause:

1. Alleviating hot flashes and night sweats.

2. Managing mood swings and irritability.

3. Addressing vaginal dryness and enhancing sexual health.

4. Aiding in weight management and reducing bloating.

To guide you, I've immersed myself in studies focused solely on human trials, setting aside theoretical or animal-based research. The goal? To highlight supplements that promise relief and have shown tangible results. It's essential to remember that while a supplement may rank high on this list, it doesn't guarantee unparalleled effectiveness. It simply means there's compelling evidence backing its benefits.

Let's begin our exploration:

Calcium

The post-menopausal hormonal decline can escalate bone deterioration. Ensuring sufficient calcium intake is pivotal. Women below 51 should aim for 1,000 milligrams daily, while those aged 51 and above should target 1,200 milligrams.

Tip: Prioritize dietary sources for your calcium intake. Opt for modest doses paired with meals throughout the day (limited to 500 mg per serving) if supplements become necessary for optimal absorption.

Vitamin D

Vitamin D plays a crucial role in bone health, standing shoulder to shoulder with calcium. It's the bridge that enables our body to absorb calcium effectively. The general recommendation is 600 IU daily for adults, while those above 70 should aim for 800 IU. While food and supplements offer good sources of Vitamin D, the sun is nature's original provider.

Tip: While sunlight can help our skin produce Vitamin D, even brief exposure can harm the skin. Thus, it's wiser to prioritise dietary sources and consider supplements if your intake is insufficient.

Wild Yam

Wild yam-derived pills and creams are often touted as natural substitutes for hormone therapy during menopause. These yams contain compounds bearing a resemblance to estrogen and progesterone. However, it's uncertain whether these compounds are bioactive in humans. Clinical research to date hasn't conclusively demonstrated their efficacy in alleviating menopausal symptoms.

Soy Isoflavones

Women undergoing menopause in the U.S. experience hot flashes at a rate eight times higher than their counterparts in Asian countries. Might the prevalent soy consumption in Asian diets be a key differentiator? It's a plausible theory. Research indicates that soy can moderately alleviate hot flashes symptoms. Clinical investigations highlight that introducing soy protein with diverse isoflavone concentrations may diminish the frequency and severity of hot flashes, especially for those enduring them frequently. Moreover, soy isoflavones could serve as a buffer against mood swings and depressive episodes, and while they might offer relief from vaginal dryness, outcomes differ from one study to another.

Black Cohosh

Derived from the Actaea racemosa plant, black cohosh can provide moderate relief from menopausal symptoms, particularly hot flashes. It's best to opt for standardised commercial extracts to get optimal results.

St. John's Wort

St. John's Wort is an herbal derivative from the Hypericum perforatum plant, renowned for its mood-elevating properties. Research suggests that it can be as effective as some mood medications. It can also reduce the frequency and severity of hot flashes, enhancing overall well-being during menopause.

Vitex Agnus-Castus (Chasteberry)

Derived from the chaste tree fruit, research indicates that chasteberry extract may relieve specific menopausal symptoms like hot flashes and potentially reduce anxiety and related symptoms.

Evening Primrose Oil

Often hailed for its potential skin and hormonal benefits, this oil might offer some relief from mood-related symptoms of menopause. However, its efficacy in treating typical menopausal symptoms remains unclear.

Sage

Beyond its culinary uses, sage, derived from the Salvia officinalis plant, has shown promise in alleviating specific menopausal symptoms like hot flashes, sleep disturbances, and fatigue. Yet, the focus is primarily on standardised commercial extracts, leaving the potential of the general herb ambiguous.

Royal Jelly

Produced by bees for their queen, royal jelly has been linked to some health benefits. While a few studies hint at its potential for relieving menopausal symptoms, more research is needed to establish its definitive role.

Red Clover

Though it contains beneficial isoflavones, research on red clover presents a mixed bag. Some studies show mild benefits, especially when paired with other supplements, but the quality and funding sources of these studies are worth noting.

Flaxseed

Recognised for potential weight loss effects in overweight menopausal women, flaxseed might also offer relief from hot flashes and night sweats. However, its unique benefits are still debated, with some studies suggesting other grains could provide similar results.

Panax Ginseng

Korean red ginseng, in particular, has shown the potential to enhance sexual arousal and satisfaction in postmenopausal women. However, its impact on other menopausal symptoms remains inconsistent.

DHEA

After age 30, our body's natural DHEA levels, dubbed the youth hormone, begin to decline. Some preliminary studies suggest that DHEA supplements might help alleviate menopausal symptoms like reduced libido and hot flashes. However, the results are inconclusive, as other research has found no significant benefits. It's worth noting that there are concerns regarding extended use or high doses of DHEA potentially increasing the risk of breast cancer.

When contemplating supplements for menopause, it's essential to align choices with your unique symptoms. Focusing on bone health with vitamin D and calcium may suffice for those lucky enough to have minimal symptoms. However, if you're grappling with challenges like hot flashes, a combination of supplements, such as soy isoflavones and black cohosh, might be beneficial. Consulting with a healthcare professional before starting any new regimen is always recommended.

Navigating menopause is about understanding the changes and finding the right tools to ease the journey. While supplements can be part of the solution, always consult a healthcare professional before introducing any new regimen.

Remember that the rankings presented are based on the quality and volume of research behind each supplement, not necessarily their efficacy for every individual. Instead of flooding your system with multiple supplements, it's wiser to handpick 2 or 3 that align with the specific challenges you're facing during menopause. For example, combining soy isoflavones and St. John's wort might be beneficial if you're navigating mood fluctuations and hot flashes. If vaginal dryness is a concern, consider integrating Panax ginseng into your routine. Beyond supplements, never underestimate the power of a balanced diet and consistent exercise, especially when maintaining a healthy weight. Solely leaning on supplements for menopausal relief isn't the most holistic strategy. I aim to arm you with evidence-based insights to make informed choices tailored to your menopausal journey.

Chapter 16
Mindful Menopause

The Interplay of Hormones and Emotion

Women's lives are punctuated by hormonal changes from the start of menstruation to the end of menopause. As women approach menopause, typically in their late 40s to early 60s, they may experience physiological and psychological shifts. It's a transformative period, marked by the cessation of menstruation, but it's also a phase of introspection, growth, and, at times, mental unrest.

Mood Fluctuations and Menopause

The hormonal imbalances associated with menopause, particularly the decline in oestrogen levels, can influence neurotransmitters in the brain such as serotonin and dopamine. This can lead to mood swings, irritability, sadness, or even depression. While many women transition through menopause smoothly, others might find it challenging due to these emotional fluctuations.

Anxiety and Stress

Some women report heightened anxiety during the menopausal transition. This can be due to hormonal shifts and life stressors typical of midlife, such as caregiving for ageing parents, health changes, or reevaluating life goals. Recognising the source of this anxiety is the first step to addressing it.

The Power of Recognition and Intervention

Awareness is crucial. Understanding menopause can influence mental health can empower women to seek help when they feel emotionally off-balance. Interventions can be as simple as lifestyle changes, such as incorporating regular exercise, which boosts mood. Mindfulness practices, such as meditation or yoga, can also be beneficial.

For those who experience profound mood disturbances, seeking professional help is essential. Cognitive-behavioural therapy (CBT) has proven effective in helping many navigate the emotional challenges of menopause. Cognitive Behavioral Therapy, commonly known as CBT, is a form of psychotherapy grounded in the belief that our thoughts, feelings, and behaviours are intricately connected. CBT aims to bring about positive changes in one's emotional state and actions by identifying and addressing negative thought patterns and behaviours. For women navigating the tumultuous waters of menopause, CBT can be a lighthouse. Emotional and physical changes, such as mood swings, hot flashes, sleep disturbances, and feelings of anxiety or depression, often accompany the menopausal transition. These can sometimes be exacerbated by ingrained negative beliefs or self-talk about ageing and femininity.

Engaging in CBT can empower women during this transition. By recognising and challenging these negative thought patterns, women can develop more adaptive ways of thinking and responding to their symptoms. For instance, CBT can equip women with strategies to manage hot flash triggers or cope with sleep disturbances, improving overall well-being. CBT offers a practical and solution-focused approach, providing women with the tools they need to sail through menopause with resilience and a positive mindset.

Hormone Replacement Therapy (HRT) can also be a solution for some. However, it's essential to note that while HRT offers several benefits, it also comes with potential risks, such as increased blood clots, stroke, and certain types of cancer. Therefore, the decision to start HRT should be made on an individual basis, taking into account the woman's overall health, the severity of her symptoms, and her personal preferences. Discuss the pros and cons of HRT with your healthcare provider; they can help assess whether it's a suitable option for you and provide a prescription if deemed appropriate.

Community and Connection

One of the most powerful tools for mental wellness during menopause is connection. Sharing experiences with peers can provide solace and understanding. Support groups, either in person or online, can be a safe space for women to discuss their feelings and offer mutual support

I recently hopped on the Substack platform, "Letters from Love", curated by the iconic Elizabeth Gilbert, best known for "Eat, Pray, Love". Over two decades ago, Elizabeth began penning letters to herself from a viewpoint of unwavering love. This transformative habit ushered in a wave of peace, self-appreciation, and compassion for her. Often, we become our harshest judge, making me wonder why I hadn't embraced this practice sooner. The platform encourages us to integrate this ritual into our daily lives, fostering a bond with unconditional love. We frequently seek such love externally, overlooking the first place we should find it — within us. If you want to join me, you can find Elizabeth's project here at https://elizabethgilbert.substack.com.

One final word

As the last page of this book turns, I want every reader, especially each woman journeying through her menopause phase, to pause and reflect. Menopause isn't merely a phase; it's an epoch, an era of transformation. A phase when the universe whispers to you, reminding you of your strength, resilience, and the countless seasons you've weathered.

Remember the first time you felt a flutter in your womb, the challenges of childbirth, or the powerful surge of emotions only you could understand? As you tread this new path, know it's a rite of passage – a journey from one phase of wisdom to another.

While society often paints menopause as an ending, I see it as a poignant beginning. It's a time to embrace the essence of who you truly are, to celebrate every wrinkle, every emotion, and every memory. It's an opportunity to be mindful, to listen to your body's symphony, and to dance to its ever-changing rhythms.

So here's to every hot flash, every restless night, and every new beginning. Here's to celebrating the beautiful tapestry of life, woven with threads of experiences, memories, and lessons. Here's to you, the resilient woman standing tall with the wisdom of the past and the promise of the future.

Let the sunset of menopause be not an end but a dazzling horizon of hope, growth, and unbridled love for yourself.

Chapter 17
References

Skeaff CM, Miller J. Dietary fat and coronary heart disease: summary of evidence from prospective cohort and randomised controlled trials. Ann Nutr Metab. 2009;55(1-3):173-201. doi: 10.1159/000229002. Epub 2009 Sep 15. PMID: 19752542.

Siri-Tarino PW, Sun Q, Hu FB, Krauss RM. Meta-analysis of prospective cohort studies evaluating the association of saturated fat with cardiovascular disease. Am J Clin Nutr. 2010 Mar;91(3):535-46. doi: 10.3945/ajcn.2009.27725. Epub 2010 Jan 13. PMID: 20071648; PMCID: PMC2824152.

Chowdhury R, Warnakula S, Kunutsor S, Crowe F, Ward HA, Johnson L, Franco OH, Butterworth AS, Forouhi NG, Thompson SG, Khaw KT, Mozaffarian D, Danesh J, Di Angelantonio E. Association of dietary, circulating, and supplement fatty acids with coronary risk: a systematic review and meta-analysis. Ann Intern Med. 2014 Mar 18;160(6):398-406. doi: 10.7326/M13-1788. Erratum in: Ann Intern Med. 2014 May 6;160(9):658. PMID: 24723079.

Mahmood SS, Levy D, Vasan RS, Wang TJ. The Framingham Heart Study and the epidemiology of cardiovascular disease: a historical perspective. Lancet. 2014 Mar 15;383(9921):999-1008. doi: 10.1016/S0140-6736(13)61752-3. Epub 2013 Sep 29. PMID: 24084292; PMCID: PMC4159698.

Frantz ID Jr, Dawson EA, Ashman PL, Gatewood LC, Bartsch GE, Kuba K, Brewer ER. Test of effect of lipid lowering by diet on cardiovascular risk. The Minnesota Coronary Survey. Arteriosclerosis. 1989 Jan-Feb;9(1):129-35. doi: 10.1161/01.atv.9.1.129. PMID: 2643423.

Ramsden CE, Zamora D, Majchrzak-Hong S, Faurot KR, Broste SK, Frantz RP, Davis JM, Ringel A, Suchindran CM, Hibbeln JR. Re-evaluation of the traditional diet-heart hypothesis: analysis of recovered data from Minnesota Coronary Experiment (1968-73). BMJ. 2016 Apr 12;353:i1246. doi: 10.1136/bmj.i1246. PMID: 27071971; PMCID: PMC4836695.

Prentice RL, Caan B, Chlebowski RT, et al. Low-fat dietary pattern and risk of invasive breast cancer: the Women's Health Initiative Randomized Controlled Dietary Modification Trial. JAMA. 2006; 295:629-42.

Beresford SA, Johnson KC, Ritenbaugh C, et al. Low-fat dietary pattern and risk of colorectal cancer: the Women's Health Initiative Randomized Controlled Dietary Modification Trial. JAMA.2006; 295:643-54.

Howard BV, Van Horn L, Hsia J, et al. Low-fat dietary pattern and risk of cardiovascular disease: the Women's Health Initiative Randomized Controlled Dietary Modification Trial. JAMA. 2006; 295:655-66.

Howard BV, Manson JE, Stefanick ML, et al. Low-fat dietary pattern and weight change over 7 years: the Women's Health Initiative Dietary Modification Trial. JAMA. 2006; 295:39-49.

Michels KB, Willett WC. The women's health initiative: will it resolve the issues? Recent Results in Cancer Research. 1996; 140:295-305.

Prentice RL, Sheppard L. Dietary fat and cancer: consistency of the epidemiologic data, and disease prevention that may follow from a practical reduction in fat consumption. Cancer Causes and Contr ol.1990; 1:81-97; discussion 99-109.

Prentice RL, Sheppard L. Dietary fat and cancer: rejoinder and discussion of research strategies. Cancer Causes and Control. 1991; 2:53-8.

Willett WC, Stampfer MJ. Dietary fat and cancer: another view? Cancer Causes and Control. 1990; 1:103-109.

Multiple risk factor intervention trial. Risk factor changes and mortality results. Multiple Risk Factor Intervention Trial Research Group. JAMA. 1982; 248:1465-77.

Willett W. Nutritional epidemiology. New York: Oxford University Press, 1998.

Persky VW, Kempthorne-Rawson J, Shekelle RB. Personality and risk of cancer: 20-year follow-up of the Western Electric Study. Psychosom Med. 1987 Sep-Oct;49(5):435-49. doi: 10.1097/00006842 -198709000-00001. PMID: 3671633.

Grundy SM, D'Agostino RB Sr, Mosca L, Burke GL, Wilson PW, Rader DJ, Cleeman JI, Roccella EJ, Cutler JA, Friedman LM. Cardiovascular risk assessment based on US cohort studies: findings from a National Heart, Lung, and Blood institute workshop. Circulation. 2001 Jul 24;104(4):491-6. doi: 10.1161/01.cir.104.4.491. PMID: 11468215.

Kearns CE, Schmidt LA, Glantz SA. Sugar Industry and Coronary Heart Disease Research: A Historical Analysis of Internal Industry Documents. JAMA Intern Med. 2016 Nov 1;176(11):1680-1685. doi: 10.1001/jamainternmed.2016.5394. Erratum in: JAMA Intern Med. 2016 Nov 1;176(11):1729. PMID: 27617709; PMCID: PMC5099084.

Kalm, L., & Semba, R., (2005). They starved so that others be better fed: Remembering Ancel keys and the Minnesota experiment. Journal of Nutrition, 135 1347-1352.

Keys, A., Brozek, J., Henschel, A., Mickelsen, O., & Taylor, H. L. (1950). The Biology of Human Starvation (2 Vols.). University of Minnesota Press, Minneapolis, MN.

Gardner CD, Kiazand A, Alhassan S, Kim S, Stafford RS, Balise RR, Kraemer HC, King AC. Comparison of the Atkins, Zone, Ornish, and LEARN diets for change in weight and related risk factors among overweight premenopausal women: the A TO Z Weight Loss Study: a randomized trial. JAMA. 2007 Mar 7;297(9):969-77. doi: 1 0.1001/jama.297.9.969. Erratum in: JAMA. 2007 Jul 11;298(2):178. PMID: 17341711.

Phinney SD. Ketogenic diets and physical performance. Nutr Metab (Lond). 2004 Aug 17;1(1):2. doi: 10.1186/1743-7075-1-2 . PMID: 15507148; PMCID: PMC524027.

Henry, R.R., Gumbiner, B., Ditzler, T., Wallace, P., Lyon, R., & Glauber, H.S. (1993). Intensive conventional insulin therapy for type II diabetes. Metabolic effects during a 6-mo outpatient trial. Diabetes Care1993 Jan;16(1):21-31. doi: 10.2337/diacare.16.1.21.

Fielding BA, Frayn KN. Lipoprotein lipase and the disposition of dietary fatty acids. Br J Nutr. 1998 Dec;80(6):495-502. doi: 10.1017 /s0007114598001585. PMID: 10211047.

Liu, D., Huang, Y., Huang, C., Yang, S., Wei, X., Zhang, P., Guo, D., Lin, J., Xu, B., Li, C., He, H., He, J., Liu, S., Shi, L., Xue, Y., Zhang, H. (2022). Calorie Restriction with or without Time-Restricted Eating in Weight Loss. New England Journal of Medicine, 386(16), 1495-1504. doi: 10.1056/NEJMoa2114833.

Cienfuegos S, Gabel K, Kalam F, Ezpeleta M, Wiseman E, Pavlou V, Lin S, Oliveira ML, Varady KA. Effects of 4- and 6-h Time-Restricted Feeding on Weight and Cardiometabolic Health: A Randomized Controlled Trial in Adults with Obesity. Cell Metab. 2020 Sep 1;32 (3):366-378.e3. doi: 10.1016/j.cmet.2020.06.018. Epub 2020 Jul 15. PMID: 32673591; PMCID: PMC9407646.

Phinney SD. Ketogenic diets and physical performance. Nutr Metab (Lond). 2004 Aug 17;1(1):2. doi: 10.1186/1743-7075-1-2 . PMID: 15507148; PMCID: PMC524027.

Phinney SD, Horton ES, Sims EA, Hanson JS, Danforth E Jr, LaGrange BM. Capacity for moderate exercise in obese subjects after adaptation to a hypocaloric, ketogenic diet. J Clin Invest. 1980 Nov;66(5):1152-61. doi: 10.1172/JCI109945. PMID: 7000826; PMCID: PMC371554.

Moro T, Tinsley G, Bianco A, Marcolin G, Pacelli QF, Battaglia G, Palma A, Gentil P, Neri M, Paoli A. Effects of eight weeks of time-restricted feeding (16/8) on basal metabolism, maximal strength, body composition, inflammation, and cardiovascular risk factors in resistance-trained males. J Transl Med. 2016 Oct 13;14(1):290. doi: 10.1186/s12967-016-1044-0. PMID: 27737674; PMCID: PMC5064803.

Cherif A, Roelands B, Meeusen R, Chamari K. Effects of Intermittent Fasting, Caloric Restriction, and Ramadan Intermittent Fasting on Cognitive Performance at Rest and During Exercise in Adults. Sports Med. 2016 Jan;46(1):35-47. doi: 10.1007/s40279-015-0408 -6. PMID: 26438184.

Hall KD. Energy compensation and metabolic adaptation: "The Biggest Loser" study reinterpreted. Obesity (Silver Spring). 2022 Jan;30(1):11-13. doi: 10.1002/oby.23308. Epub 2021 Nov 23. PMID: 34816627.

Fanti M, Mishra A, Longo VD, Brandhorst S. Time-Restricted Eating, Intermittent Fasting, and Fasting-Mimicking Diets in Weight

Loss. Curr Obes Rep. 2021 Jun;10(2):70-80. doi: 10.1007/s13679-021-00424-2. Epub 2021 Jan 29. PMID: 33512641.

Cahill GF Jr, Aoki TT, Ruderman NB. Ketosis. Trans Am Clin Climatol Assoc. 1973;84:184-202. PMID: 4199621; PMCID: PMC2441301.

Cahill GF Jr. Starvation in man. N Engl J Med. 1970 Mar 19;282(12):668-75. doi: 10.1056/NEJM197003192821209. PMID: 4915800.

Liu D, Huang Y, Huang C, Yang S, Wei X, Zhang P, Guo D, Lin J, Xu B, Li C, He H, He J, Liu S, Shi L, Xue Y, Zhang H. Calorie Restriction with or without Time-Restricted Eating in Weight Loss. N Engl J Med. 2022 Apr 21;386(16):1495-1504. doi: 10.1056/NEJMoa2114833. PMID: 35443107.

The Diabetes Control And Complications Trial Research Group. Influence of intensive diabetes treatment on body weight and composition of adults with type 1 diabetes in the Diabetes Control and Complications Trial. Diabetes Care. 2001 Oct;24(10):1711-21. doi: 10.2337/diacare.24.10.1711. PMID: 11574431; PMCID: PMC2663516.

Wilding JPH, Batterham RL, Calanna S, Davies M, Van Gaal LF, Lingvay I, McGowan BM, Rosenstock J, Tran MTD, Wadden TA, Wharton S, Yokote K, Zeuthen N, Kushner RF; STEP 1 Study Group. Once-Weekly Semaglutide in Adults with Overweight or Obesity. N Engl J Med. 2021 Mar 18;384(11):989-1002. doi: 10.1056/NEJMoa2032183. Epub 2021 Feb 10. PMID: 33567185.

Natalucci G, Riedl S, Gleiss A, Zidek T, Frisch H. Spontaneous 24-h ghrelin secretion pattern in fasting subjects: maintenance of a meal-related pattern. Eur J Endocrinol. 2005 Jun;152(6):845-50. doi: 10.1530/eje.1.01919. PMID: 15941923.

Catenacci VA, Pan Z, Ostendorf D, Brannon S, Gozansky WS, Mattson MP, Martin B, MacLean PS, Melanson EL, Troy Donahoo W. A randomized pilot study comparing zero-calorie alternate-day fasting to daily caloric restriction in adults with obesity. Obesity (Silver Spring). 2016 Sep;24(9):1874-83. doi: 10.1002/oby.21581. PMID: 27569118; PMCID: PMC5042570.

Patel JN, Coppack SW, Goldstein DS, Miles JM, Eisenhofer G. Norepinephrine spillover from human adipose tissue before and after a 72-hour fast. J Clin Endocrinol Metab. 2002 Jul;87(7):3373-7. doi: 10.1210/jcem.87.7.8695. PMID: 12107252.

Brunetti P. La terapia insulinica [Insulin therapy]. Minerva Endocrinol. 2001 Jun;26(2):65-86. Italian. PMID: 11479436.

Hendrix, Jennifer & Aikens, James & Saslow, Laura. (2019). Dietary Weight Loss Strategies for Self and Patients: A Cross-Sectional survey of Female Physicians. Obesity Medicine. 17. 100158. 10.101 6/j.obmed.2019.100158.

Schaumberg K, Anderson DA, Reilly EE, Anderson LM. Does short-term fasting promote pathological eating patterns? Eat Behav. 2015 Dec;19:168-72. doi: 10.1016/j.eatbeh.2015.09.005. Epub 2015 Sep 24. PMID: 26431904.

Johnstone AM, Faber P, Gibney ER, Elia M, Horgan G, Golden BE, Stubbs RJ. Effect of an acute fast on energy compensation and feeding behaviour in lean men and women. Int J Obes Relat Metab Disord. 2002 Dec;26(12):1623-8. doi: 10.1038/sj.ijo.080215 1. PMID: 12461679.

Berin E, Hammar M, Lindblom H, Lindh-Åstrand L, Spetz Holm AC. Effects of resistance training on quality of life in postmenopausal women with vasomotor symptoms. Climacteric. 2022 Jun;25(3):264-270. doi: 10.1080/13697137.2021.1941849 . Epub 2021 Jul 9. PMID: 34240669.

Khalafi M, Sakhaei MH, Habibi Maleki A, Rosenkranz SK, Pourvaghar MJ, Fang Y, Korivi M. Influence of exercise type and duration on cardiorespiratory fitness and muscular strength in post-menopausal women: a systematic review and meta-analysis. Front Cardiovasc Med. 2023 May 9;10:1190187. doi: 10.3389/fcv m.2023.1190187. PMID: 37229231; PMCID: PMC10204927.

Writing Group for the Women's Health Initiative Investigators, including Jacques E. Rossouw, MD; Garnet L. Anderson, PhD; Ross L. Prentice, PhD; Andrea Z. LaCroix, PhD; Charles Kooperberg, PhD; Marcia L. Stefanick, PhD; et al. "Risks and Benefits of Estrogen Plus Progestin in Healthy Postmenopausal Women: Principal Results from the Women's Health Initiative Randomized Controlled Trial." In: Journal of the American Medical Association (JAMA), Volume 288, Issue 3, pages 321-333, 2002.

The Women's Health Initiative Steering Committee, including Andrea Z. LaCroix, PhD; Rowan T. Chlebowski, MD; Marcia L. Stefanick, PhD; JoAnn E. Manson, MD; Aaron K. Aragaki, MS; et al. "Effects of Conjugated Equine Estrogen in Postmenopausal Women with Hysterectomy: The Women's Health Initiative Randomized Controlled Trial." In: Journal of the American Medical Association (JAMA), Volume 291, Issue 14, pages 1701-1712, 2004.

Lee CG, Carr MC, Murdoch SJ, et al. Adipokines, inflammation, and visceral adiposity across the menopausal transition: a prospective study. The Journal of Clinical Endocrinology & Metabolism. 2009 Apr;94(4):1104-10. doi: 10.1210/jc.2008-0701.

Franklin RM, Ploutz-Snyder L, Kanaley JA. Longitudinal changes in abdominal fat distribution with menopause. Metabolism 2009 Mar;58(3):311-5. doi: 10.1016/j.metabol.2008.09.030.

Maffei L, Murata Y, Rochira V, et al. Dysmetabolic syndrome in a man with a novel mutation of the aromatase gene: Effects of testosterone, alendronate, and estradiol treatment. The Journal of Clinical Endocrinology & Metabolism. 2004 Jan;89(1):61-70. doi: 10.1210/jc.2003-030313.

San-Millán I, Brooks GA. Assessment of Metabolic Flexibility by Means of Measuring Blood Lactate, Fat, and Carbohydrate Oxidation Responses to Exercise in Professional Endurance Athletes and Less-Fit Individuals. Sports Med. 2018 Feb;48(2):467-479. doi: 10.1007/s40 279-017-0751-x. PMID: 28623613.

San-Millán I, Stefanoni D, Martinez JL, Hansen KC, D'Alessandro A, Nemkov T. Metabolomics of Endurance Capacity in World Tour Professional Cyclists. Front Physiol. 2020 Jun 5;11:578. doi: 10.338 9/fphys.2020.00578. PMID: 32581847; PMCID: PMC7291837.

Bonds DE, Lasser N, Qi L, et al. The effect of conjugated equine oestrogen on diabetes incidence: the Women's Health Initiative randomised trial. Diabetologia. 2006 Mar;49(3):459-68. doi: 10.1007/s 00125-005-0096-0.

Margolis KL, Bonds DE, Rodabough RJ, et al. Effect of oestrogen plus progestin on the incidence of diabetes in postmenopausal women: results from the Women's Health Initiative Hormone Trial. Diabetologia. 2004 Jul;47(7):1175-87. doi: 10.1007/s00125-004-14 48-x.

Sá KMM, da Silva GR, Martins UK, Colovati MES, Crizol GR, Riera R, Pacheco RL, Martimbianco ALC. Resistance training for postmenopausal women: systematic review and meta-analysis. Menopause. 2023 Jan 1;30(1):108-116. doi: 10.1097/GME.000000 0000002079. Epub 2022 Oct 25. PMID: 36283059.

Rossouw JE, Anderson GL, Prentice RL, LaCroix AZ, Kooperberg C, Stefanick ML, Jackson RD, Beresford SA, Howard BV, Johnson KC, Kotchen JM, Ockene J; Writing Group for the Women's Health Initiative Investigators. Risks and benefits of estrogen plus progestin in healthy postmenopausal women: principal results From the Women's Health Initiative randomized controlled trial. JAMA. 2002 Jul 17;288(3):321-33. doi: 10.1001/jama.288.3.321. PMID: 12117397.

Melnyk BM, Kelly SA, Stephens J, Dhakal K, McGovern C, Tucker S, Hoying J, McRae K, Ault S, Spurlock E, Bird SB. Interventions to Improve Mental Health, Well-Being, Physical Health, and Lifestyle Behaviors in Physicians and Nurses: A Systematic Review. Am J Health Promot. 2020 Nov;34(8):929-941. doi: 10.1177/08 90117120920451. Epub 2020 Apr 27. PMID: 32338522; PMCID: PMC8982669.

Fights SD. Nurses' Health Study. Medsurg Nurs. 2011 Jan-Feb;20(1):5, 44. PMID: 21446287.

Chen LR, Chen KH. Utilization of Isoflavones in Soybeans for Women with Menopausal Syndrome: An Overview. Int J Mol Sci. 2021 Mar 22;22(6):3212. doi: 10.3390/ijms22063212. PMID: 33809928; PMCID: PMC8004126.

Chan SW. Panax ginseng, Rhodiola rosea and Schisandra chinensis. Int J Food Sci Nutr. 2012 Mar;63 Suppl 1:75-81. doi: 10.3109/096 37486.2011.627840. Epub 2011 Nov 1. PMID: 22039930.

Hyun SH, Kim SW, Seo HW, Youn SH, Kyung JS, Lee YY, In G, Park CK, Han CK. Physiological and pharmacological features of the non-saponin components in Korean Red Ginseng. J Ginseng Res. 2020 Jul;44(4):527-537. doi: 10.1016/j.jgr.2020.01.005. Epub 2020 Feb 6. PMID: 32617032; PMCID: PMC7322739.

Rabijewski M, Papierska L, Binkowska M, Maksym R, Jankowska K, Skrzypulec-Plinta W, Zgliczynski W. Supplementation of dehydroepiandrosterone (DHEA) in pre- and postmenopausal women - position statement of expert panel of Polish Menopause and An-

dropause Society. Ginekol Pol. 2020;91(9):554-562. doi: 10.5603/G
P.2020.0091. PMID: 33030737.

Afterword

In the heart of Singapore, amidst the bustle of clinics and the hum of urban life, I've borne witness to a journey shared by countless women. From the patient rooms to my own home, the tapestry of womanhood is rich with stories of strength, resilience, and transformation.

As a daughter, I've seen the women who came before me grapple with the silent shifts of menopause, their experiences often whispered in hushed tones, veiled by societal expectations. As a mother, I carry forward their legacy, aiming to instil in the next generation a deeper understanding and appreciation for the myriad phases of a woman's life.

Navigating the male-dominated realm of the medical profession has sharpened my resolve to advocate for women's health, especially when it concerns the complexities of menopause. Each patient I meet isn't just a case study but a testament to the incredible strength that women possess. They inspire me daily with their grace, humour, and tenacity, even when faced with the challenges of ageing in a world that often seems indifferent to their struggles.

"Get Your Sexy Back" is more than just a book; it's a tribute to every woman who has ever felt overshadowed or misunderstood. It's a call to embrace our bodies, our journeys, and our stories. It's an invitation to find power in vulnerability, beauty in the scars, and grace in the midst of change.

To every woman reading this – whether you're a daughter, a mother, or walking the path of menopause – know that you are seen, you are valued, and you are not alone. Together, we forge a new narrative, one that celebrates the multifaceted beauty of womanhood.

With heartfelt gratitude and unwavering solidarity,

Chai Ling

About the Author

Dr. Low Chai Ling, a distinguished alumna of King's College, London, and Cardiff University, is a trailblazer in the world of aesthetic medicine. Graduating from the prestigious Guy's & St Thomas's Hospital, Dr. Low began her pioneering journey by venturing into the then-infant realm of aesthetic medicine in Beverly Hills during the late 90s.

In 2003, her vision materialised as she founded The Sloane Clinic, one of Singapore's pioneering aesthetic clinics. Determined to evolve her aesthetic vision without boundaries, she later established SW1 Clinic. This endeavour not only symbolised her aesthetic journey's evolution but also gave rise to one of Singapore's most prominent aesthetic, plastic surgery, and medical spa centres. SW1's inception drew inspiration from Dr. Low's student days in the Royal Borough of Kensington & Chelsea, encapsulating her 14-year transformative journey in the field.

Known for her keen aesthetic eye and unmatched medical expertise, Dr. Low is also an accomplished author. Her works, including "In Full Bloom: Look Fabulous During and After Pregnancy," grace bookshelves worldwide. Beyond her clinics, she has significantly impacted the global aesthetic community as a master trainer, speaker, and key opinion leader.

However, her journey isn't solely about aesthetics. At the heart of Dr. Low's endeavours is a commitment to empowering individuals. From conceptualising SW1 treatments reflecting the spirit of iconic women to launching GLOW UP, an initiative aimed at boosting teenagers' self-confidence, she believes in a holistic approach to beauty and wellness.

Her dedication extends beyond her profession. Actively championing causes for the disadvantaged, Dr. Low fervently believes in empowering women to drive societal change. Committed to creating a compassionate society, she generously contributes a portion of her personal and clinic income towards myriad social causes.

Esteemed by celebrities across Asia, Dr. Low's patient-first approach, combined with her desire to inspire and educate, makes her a beacon in the integration of wellness and beauty.